'*Honey Blood* is one of the most exuberant, life-affirming memoirs I have ever read. The fact that it is about the uncompromising reality of childhood cancer makes it all the more extraordinary. Read it and be utterly bowled over by Kirsty Everett's astonishing courage, honesty and cheeky humour.'

— Patti Miller, author

'Do not be afraid of this book. The big C in it is not cancer, it's courage. The courage to deal with pain, loss, fear and the shattering of a young girl's big dreams.

'Instead of tiptoeing around the tough stuff, and leaving the most difficult bits out, Kirsty Everett dives right in, taking the reader into her world, bravely, honestly, with raw humour and grit. We get up close to her tight-knit family, boisterous friends, tender first loves, doctors both brusque and kind, and rude strangers. Death hovers on every page, but life's vitality and Kirsty's defiant spirit shove it aside.

'This refreshingly straight-talking account of adolescent leukaemia goes beyond pain to a fuller, wiser, deeper understanding of what really matters when everything you hope for hangs by a thread. It offers the best medicine for anyone who has ever faced the relentless physical and mental odds and obstacles that create seemingly insurmountable roadblocks as tests of character. It may not be a cure, but it is one mighty transfusion of the powerful drugs that make us human and help us survive: hope, compassion, and love.'

— Caroline Baum, author

Honey Blood

Kirsty Everett

HarperCollins*Publishers*

HarperCollins*Publishers*
Australia • Brazil • Canada • France • Germany • Holland • India
Italy • Japan • Mexico • New Zealand • Poland • Spain • Sweden
Switzerland • United Kingdom • United States of America

HarperCollins acknowledges the Traditional Custodians
of the lands upon which we live and work, and pays respect
to Elders past and present.

First published on Gadigal Country in Australia in 2020
by HarperCollins*Publishers* Australia Pty Limited
ABN 36 009 913 517
harpercollins.com.au

A catalogue record for this book is available from the National Library of Australia.

ISBN 978 1 4607 6664 4 (paperback)
ISBN 978 1 4607 1258 0 (ebook)

Cover design by Amy Daoud, HarperCollins Design Studio
Cover image by Orlova Maria at Unsplash
Typeset in Bembo Std by Kirby Jones
Unless otherwise credited, all photos are from the collection of Kirsty Everett

Printed and bound by CPI Group (UK) Ltd, Croydon, CR0 4YY

For Peter James Everett and Benjamin Malesev —
the truly good men.

And for all the young people who are no longer alive because cancer
stole them away from their families. There's not enough room in my
locket for all of you, but you have a permanent place in my heart.

CONTENTS

CHAPTER 1

It's *Only* a Day

'Oh good, Kirsty's here! Wait until you see her curl up and do this cold turkey.'

They called it 'Day Only', meaning you only spent the day there having treatment. 'Day Only' consisted of one large room at the very end of a hospital ward. I don't know why they didn't let us all spread out and have one room each, because every other room on this ward was now empty and unused. Perhaps they wanted to keep all of us cancer kids in the one place.

Day Only had eight beds, seven of which were proper single beds. Six of those beds had bald children in them, which meant the seventh bed was for me. The eighth bed — the bed near the door — was the treatment bed. This was the altar where our innocence was sacrificed to the cancer gods. This wasn't so much a bed as a hard padded bench that was just like a large ironing board. Next to it was a privacy curtain that they could pull around the bed whenever a patient was placed upon it.

I sat down on the last empty bed, got out a book — *Unreal* by Paul Jennings — and began to read. Mum plonked her handbag on the ground and pulled out the latest issue of *Women's Weekly* before sitting down in a beige chair next to me.

'Where's that lollipop for Bradley? We should get Kirsty to show Bradley how this gets done.'

The nurse speaking was called Karen. Karen was always here. She had long straggly hair that was a greasy tangled mess on each side of her face. Mum often said it looked like it needed a 'good wash and blow-dry'. Karen had an enormous bottom that wobbled so much that sometimes it seemed to be chasing her around the room. Karen would stride towards one of us kids and then, suddenly, her bum remembered it needed to keep up with her. She rummaged around in her pockets for a few moments and then pulled out a red lollipop. She walked over to two-year-old Bradley, who tilted his head backwards, opened his mouth wide and let out a high-pitched scream. Bradley, like all the children here, was bald. He had dark brown eyes, ghost-like skin and a frail, malnourished body. It's probably a good thing that the windows couldn't be opened because if there was a gust of wind, then Bradley would've been picked up and carried away.

His parents, like all parents at Day Only, were powerless statues.

'If you be a good boy, you can have this lollipop,' said Karen.

'I think Karen's eaten one too many lollipops,' muttered Mum to me and we had a discreet giggle at the expense of Karen's bum.

The five other children, along with Bradley, began to scream too. The choir of howling cancer children filled the room. I sat still, holding my book in my lap, and didn't make a sound. My ears began to ring and I tried to focus on the words in the book, but the cries of terror made my hands shake and the words kept jostling about.

'We'll have to do this the hard way.' Karen put the lollipop back into her pocket and motioned for another nurse to come over. As the other nurse got closer to him, Bradley's screaming became even more high-pitched. He knew what was coming. We all did. Goose bumps exploded all over my arms.

Karen tried to pick him up. He kicked and punched at her and the other nurse grabbed hold of his legs. 'Come on, Bradley,' said Karen. 'Don't be so difficult for us.'

Bradley stopped screaming for a moment, but the other children continued crying in solidarity. As he reached the treatment bed, where a registrar stood waiting for him, he wailed like he was being murdered. My ears wouldn't stop ringing. I heard a whooshing sound as the curtain was pulled around the treatment bed. We could no longer see Bradley, but we could still hear him. The other children fell silent. Bradley was on the altar now and none of us could help him.

I heard the registrar say: 'Can someone put a hand over his mouth? I can't get this needle in with him screaming like that.'

Someone covered Bradley's mouth, but I could still hear him yelling from behind the hand. Minutes ticked by. The curtain opened. Bradley had stopped screaming, but now he was sobbing as his dad carried him over to his bed and Karen wheeled Bradley's intravenous drip behind him.

'Here's your lollipop,' she chirped, as she shoved the sweet near Bradley's face. He snatched it and chucked it on the floor. 'Who's next?'

It wasn't me. They did us in order of youngest to oldest. I was ten, so I would be going last today. I would have a long time to read and listen to the shrill cries before it was my turn on the altar.

One after the other, children were taken and given their treatment. Eventually, Karen came over to my bed.

'Come on, Kirsty. Your turn.'

I swung my legs down from the bed and started to walk towards the torture table, Mum following behind me. Karen pulled a clean plastic sheet onto the bed. I used the little step next to the bed to get up onto the hard platform and immediately curled up on my side for the bone marrow biopsy, or BMA (bone marrow aspiration), which I knew they would do first.

Karen whisked the curtain around. I stared straight ahead at the curtain in front of me. Mum stood near my feet so she wouldn't be in the way, but she was always careful to position her eyes at the same spot on the curtain as I did. She didn't want to see what they needed to do to me. No one needs to see this. The curtain was bright orange with cartoon characters all over it — not Disney characters like Goofy or Donald Duck, but warped creatures that only vaguely resembled these beloved Disney characters. Red lollipops didn't make biopsies easier and neither did stupid cartoons on a curtain.

The registrar stood near me, close enough that I could now see her hands were shaking. She looked very young, like a teenager. Her face was pale white with a coating of sweat shimmering on it. Her hair was cut very short and it was spiky.

'Kirsty's different to the others,' Karen said to her. 'She won't move. This one doesn't even need anything to get through it. She does everything cold turkey.'

The registrar's eyes grew wide and she made a sort of grunting sound of disbelief.

'She's very good,' Mum chimed in. 'She knows it's important to stay very still and she doesn't like how the happy gas smells.' Between Karen and Mum, it seemed we had this registrar about forty per cent convinced of my ability to stay still while enduring agonising medical procedures. And she wasn't about to argue. Happy gas cost money. It was 1991 and sometimes Day Only didn't even have gas, so they had to use whatever they could to take the horror out of the horrifying — even if it was just a little bit. Sometimes they'd give you Pethidine, which turned the children into floppy rag dolls. If there wasn't Pethidine, then they'd give us Phenergan.

With her cold and calloused hands, Karen inched my trackpants down to expose my right hip bone to the registrar. Cold liquid was splashed across my skin, and I could feel it run down my back and create a soggy patch on the bed. The smell of antiseptic was so strong it brought water to my eyes. A small plastic sheet with a five-centimetre hole cut out of it was placed over my body as I stared at a lunatic version of Mickey Mouse. The hole was where the needle would go. The biopsy needle they were about to punch into me was silver, shiny and thick, about the same width as a plastic ink tube in the middle of a pen. To get to the bone marrow, the needle has to be pushed through the bone with great force, making it excruciatingly painful. To help with the patient's pain and anxiety, the actual slamming-in of the needle was usually done after a patient had been sedated with something, but I seemed to have earned myself a reputation of quiet endurance. I never screamed and I always stayed perfectly still, so I wasn't given anything. Step One of my treatment for today was about to begin.

The registrar hammered the needle into my hip. I blinked as the pain twanged. It felt like the sting of a wasp being administered through a bolt. Drops of bone marrow were collected in a little plastic tube, then the needle was dragged out of me slowly. It burned as it left my body. The plastic sheet with the hole in it was lifted off me. Karen splashed more antiseptic over the injection site, wiped the spot with some gauze and pressed a circle-shaped Band-Aid over the wound with her thumb.

Now it was time for Step Two, the lumbar puncture, or LP, which was my least-favourite procedure behind the curtain. A lumbar puncture is a needle into your lower spine. They collect your spinal fluid and then they inject your spine with chemo. I had to have *a lot* of these.

'Watch this,' said Karen. 'She used to be a gymnast before she got sick. That's why she can scrunch up so good.' Nobody responded.

Curling up tight for an LP is important because they need to get the needle *in between* the discs of your spine. When you stand or lie straight, all the discs in your spine squish together tightly, but when you curl up in a ball, you can create small spaces between the discs. I clutched my knees and pulled my body into the tightest ball I possibly could. The registrar began pushing on my lower spine with her icy fingers, feeling for the gap into which she would pierce the needle. Then she stopped, and Karen splashed the cold antiseptic all over my back again so that the puddle I was lying in got even bigger. Another plastic sheet with a hole in it was placed over my back. I could feel the second needle penetrate my flesh. The LP needle is not punched in like the BMA needle. It is pushed in very slowly.

It's important you don't move because if you do, you can end up with a permanent spinal injury.

'Hold her!' the registrar suddenly burst out.

'She never moves.' I heard my mum's voice coming from near my feet, but I couldn't see her. I was looking at a twisted version of Donald Duck.

The registrar ignored my mum and turned to Karen. 'Can you just hold her legs into her chest for me?'

Karen moved around to my side of the bed and pushed on my knees.

Twang!

The metal needle hit bone. The registrar had missed. She'd have to try again.

I just kept staring at the weird Donald Duck. The registrar pierced the needle again into my lower spine. It didn't get far as it slammed against bone. A banging sensation ricocheted all the way up to my neck. I didn't move. Sweat sprouted on my upper lip. The registrar had missed a second time. She'd have to keep trying until she got it in the right spot.

'She must have moved,' complained the registrar.

'Just try again,' said Karen. 'Kirsty doesn't mind if you need to have a few tries before you get it.'

I was a compact spheroid of a girl while this registrar tried again and again to get the needle into the right spot. It stung more and more each time, and each time she hit bone a horrid sensation crashed up my back. I felt cold and hot flushes all over my skin. My hearing went funny and things sounded like they had an echo. In between her attempts, I very gently wiggled my fingers and toes, as the nurses had told us to do when something hurt. My spine was on fire, but if I slightly moved my toes and fingers it refocused my brain on something else. I could not let the fire in my spine get the better of me. Twelve times this woman tried before Karen quietly suggested they get somebody else to do it.

Karen left to find someone and the registrar let out a big frustrated sigh.

'She must be moving. I never have this much trouble.' The registrar with the echidna hair stormed off.

The curtain in front of me was suddenly ripped back and a round man with rosy cheeks who smelled like he'd spilled a whole bottle of cologne on himself appeared, with Karen behind him.

'Do you mind if I have a try?' He was actually asking me.

'No, go ahead,' I said.

'I'll just have a feel first.' He pulled the plastic sheet with the hole in it off my back and pushed his warm chubby fingers into my lower spine. It throbbed terribly from the earlier failed attempts. 'I'm sorry, Kirsty, you must be very sore by now. Okay, on the count of three, we'll have one more try. One, two and three!'

On 'three', he pushed the needle in and oh boy did it sting, but it did not hit the bone.

'Got it!' He was very excited.

I exhaled. I realised I'd been holding my breath.

He counted the drops of my spinal fluid as he collected them in another small plastic tube. Then he attached a syringe filled with chemotherapy onto the needle that was still inside my spine. 'When I push in this methotrexate, it's going to feel like you're doing a wee, but I promise you will not wee on me. It just feels like you're weeing because of the pressure I'm putting on your spine when I put the medicine in. Okay?'

'Okay,' I said, familiar with the strange phenomenon.

'I'm injecting now.' An invisible foot with a large steel-capped boot trod on my bladder. My crotch surged with pins and needles. My bladder bellowed in desperation. 'And, needle is coming out in three, two, one! Okay, well done.'

Only Step Three was left. My body felt safe enough to loosen slightly. I carefully propped myself up and sat on the cancer altar with my legs hanging over the edge.

'I can put the cannula in!' The registrar came back and my body turned rigid again. 'She'd better hold still so I can find a vein.'

'All right then,' said the jolly LP guru. 'I'll leave you to it.' My shoulders and neck tightened in despair as he walked away.

Karen rolled her eyes.

'I want to put it in the back of her left hand because that's the easiest way for me to get this done.' She grabbed my wrist and squeezed it, and, with her other hand, began smacking the back of my hand to bring the veins closer to the surface.

'Kirsty's veins in her left arm have completely collapsed,' Karen said sheepishly.

'I'm sure I can get one.' The registrar gripped my wrist so tight I thought my hand might pop off. She smacked the back of my hand even harder. 'I can see a vein,' she said, and she began to 'suit up'.

When someone injects intravenous chemo into a patient, they pretty much wear a spacesuit. It's a long-sleeved gown that fully covers their whole body and their arms right down to their wrists. They put one of those medical caps over their head that looks like a shower cap. Then they put on two sets of gloves. They cover their mouth and eyes with a mask. This is because liquid chemo is like acid when it touches the skin and can literally burn your flesh. But the patient — in this case, me — doesn't get covered with anything.

The registrar slopped antiseptic onto the back of my hand and took aim with the needle. It felt like a long bee sting and immediately I knew she'd missed the vein. When a needle is safely inserted into a vein, blood will instantly begin flowing out. Nothing flowed. Heavy drops of sweat dribbled down my forehead.

'I know the vein is there,' she said. She proceeded to pull the needle backwards and forwards, trying to get it into the vein. Pain seethed under my skin. She had missed the vein, we all knew it, but none of us said anything. I didn't cry and I didn't move. I'd like to tell you that this was the only day that a registrar wasn't exactly great at their job, but this used to happen *all the time*. I don't recall any registrar ever finding a vein in my body on their first try.

The registrar swayed slightly. 'Can somebody grab a hold of this? I feel a bit dizzy.'

Karen quickly pulled on some gloves and took the needle. She was just in time as the registrar plonked down onto the floor and passed out. Other nurses came running and scooped her up and took her out of the room. As soon as the registrar was removed, Karen pulled the needle out and pushed a ball of cotton onto the wound. I was relieved to have the needle out, but I knew I still needed to have my chemo injected into a vein before I was done for the day.

Several other registrars came in, one after the other, to try to get a needle into a vein for me, but they all failed. Some tried the backs of both hands, some tried to access veins in my wrists and others tried to get veins in the middle of my arm. No one could get one and I started to wonder if they'd let me go home or not. After fourteen attempts to find a vein in my body, the round jolly man who had successfully done my lumbar puncture suddenly appeared again.

'How about we find a vein so you can go home?' he asked.

'Yes, please,' I said.

He looked at my arms and hands, which were now covered with pricks, and then his eyes ran down my legs until they settled on my feet. He picked up my right foot with his big warm hands. Using one hand, he gripped my ankle and gently tapped the top of my foot. 'I can see some thick veins in here. It will sting differently to the way it stings your arms and hands, but these veins are really good juicy ones, so I'll get the cannula in nice and quick. What do you think?'

I nodded. At this stage, I didn't care. I just wanted to have Step Three over and done with and get out of this place.

He put on the chemo spacesuit, dabbed a tiny square of antiseptic onto my foot, then said, 'One, two, three!' He pierced the needle into the top of my foot. He wasn't lying. It did sting in a different way — a far more painful way. Dark blood immediately shot out. I relished my relief. He had got the needle into the vein straight away. The stinging stopped and he attached a syringe. He injected some saline into the vein. I felt coldness flood my foot.

'I'm going to push in the vincristine,' he said. Vincristine was a drug I had had a lot of. It was clear and came in a huge syringe. 'The vincristine is going to feel cold because it has come straight out of the fridge, and as I inject it you're going to get a strong taste of metal in your mouth.' As he pressed down on the plunger, it felt like ice was spreading under my skin and my tongue hosted an explosion of saliva. It was as though I was slurping on a lozenge made of bitter orange peel.

He pulled the needle out and my body collapsed in relief and exhaustion. He put a Band-Aid on my foot and then lifted me down off the bench. 'All done! You did very well.'

'You're a legend,' I said. He laughed as he waved me goodbye.

The drive home from Day Only was a blur of discomfort as I listened to Mum sing along, out of tune, to Cher's hit song 'If I Could Turn Back Time'.

I looked at the clock on the dashboard. It was 4.37 pm. I hadn't eaten all day, but I wasn't hungry. I began to feel the chemo inside me. My insides buzzed and ached at the same time, and I felt like throwing up. I could smell the antiseptic that had been splashed all over my back, my hip and my arms. My clothes stank of the hospital.

As soon as we got home, I shuffled my way towards the couch and flopped down next to my five-year-old brother, Matthew, who was fixated on the television screen. I glanced down at my body. My hands and arms looked see-through, and the needle holes in my arms and hands and wrists were sprouting bruises. All over my tiny ten-year-old body were various shades of blues and purples and sickly-looking yellows. Every single needle hole was surrounded by its own orb of colour. I lay down on my left side, my head on a pillow and my face pointing at the Teenage Mutant Ninja Turtles who were overcoming the evil Shredder on the television. God bless the invention that is the television.

Suddenly, I could feel hot, wet snot begin to leak out of my nostrils. It was like a tap had been turned on inside my nose. I rubbed my nose with the back of my hand, but when I looked down at my hand, I saw it was covered in blood.

'Matt,' I said, 'I need tissues.'

Matthew shot up from his spot on the lounge and his brown skin turned grey as he quickly grabbed a nearby box of tissues. 'Mum!' he called out. I could hear the fear in his voice.

He kept snatching up handfuls of tissues and handing them to me, and I kept soaking them with my gigantic nosebleed. The tissues weren't enough and Matt's skin was now looking green.

Mum stuck her head in the doorway. 'Shit.' She disappeared and came back with a huge beach towel and helped me hold the towel up to my face.

Poor little Matty, I thought. *He shouldn't have to see his big sister bleeding like this.*

'It's just your platelet count dropping after chemo today,' said Mum. 'You'll probably need a platelet transfusion tomorrow.'

Matt sat with me as we waited for the nosebleed to stop, which eventually it did. They always did. I had survived another day in Day Only.

CHAPTER 2

Before

Mum's muscular arms scraped the plastic comb through my long thick hair. People told me I was a strawberry blonde, but my hair was not the same colour as strawberries.

'*My* hair used to be long like this when I was nineteen,' said Mum.

'Really? You had long hair like me?' I looked at her black short perm. I just couldn't imagine it. *My mum* with long hair. I felt like laughing as I tried to picture it.

We sat in the backyard in the morning sun, even though it was a winter's day. Mum was braiding my hair because today was an important day for me. Today I was representing the state of NSW by competing in a gymnastics competition. I'd started gymnastics at the age of four. My body was a clever combination of my mum and dad. Mum's DNA gave me my stocky strength. Dad's DNA gave me focus and dedication. My body seemed to cope with whatever demands were made of it, whether it was slipping into the splits or swinging around the bars while keeping my body in a straight line with extended arms and pointed toes. I could hold myself upside down in a handstand after all the other girls gave up and fell to the ground. I could turn cartwheel after cartwheel and launch into backflips and somersaults without feeling dizzy. It was exhilarating to do these routines, as if every particle within me could only be fully alive when I was pushing, flipping, gripping and stretching my body to its maximum capability.

I was nine years old and I wanted to be an Olympic gymnast. I wanted to be the best. I never came home from competitions without a medal, and today I had my heart set on gold.

'Ouch!' A knot. With a swift pull of the comb, Mum ripped the tangle out of existence. My scalp felt a pinch for a second. Mum made two plaits with green and gold ribbons threaded into them so my hair matched my leotard.

I looked down at my legs, hoping that the sun wasn't making new freckles. My legs looked pale and thin and they were spattered with bruises — perfectly circular stamps of blues and purples.

'It's a shame you have *those* all over your arms and legs,' said Mum, as she placed the comb next to me on the grass.

'All gymnasts get bruises. They're just from training so hard.'

Mum didn't look like she believed me. 'Have you got a headache? You look tired.' Mum's eyes were dashing all over my body. She was searching for something.

'Yes.' I wanted to lie, but she could always tell when I lied.

'The women in our family all get headaches. Hopefully you'll grow out of it,' said Mum, though she looked concerned. 'I just need to put on my shoes and then we'll be ready to go.'

She went inside, walking heavily on her heels, as she always did. I closed my eyes and pointed my face right up to the sky. For a few moments, it felt wonderful with the sun kissing my white freckly skin. I took a deep breath. Well, I tried to take a deep breath. As I inhaled, I felt like the air wasn't making it all the way into my chest. I hugged my legs and rested my head on my knees for a few moments. My headache felt like it was trying to punch a path out of my skull. *Thump, thump, thump.* With each beat of my heart, the pain in my head twanged.

I need to pull myself together.

I lifted my heavy head up and opened my eyes. My twelve-year-old brother, Brett, and Matt were sitting on the grass next to me.

'What are you doing?' asked Brett.

'Nothing. Just sitting,' I said. 'I have a headache and I'm nervous about today.'

'"I have a headache and I'm nervous about today!"' they mimicked.

'Leave me alone.'

For two boys who were so physically different — Brett with red hair and freckles, Matthew with hair as black as tar and flawless olive skin — they were annoyingly on the same wavelength when it came to pestering me.

'Leave Kirsty alone!' yelled my sixteen-year-old sister, Danielle, from the back door. Danielle was like Brett in looks, with copper hair and freckly skin, but she never harassed me and would protect me from our brothers whenever she could.

There was no time for more argument because Mum came back out. 'All right, you boys behave yourselves today,' she instructed, as we began heading towards the front of the house. 'If you're good, we can get Chinese food for dinner.'

'Yum!' exclaimed Matthew. 'Can we get honey prawns?'

'We'll see,' she said. When Mum said 'we'll see', that usually meant 'no'.

Dad gave me a hug. Dad had two hugging rules: 1) I can have one any time I like and 2) he never lets go first. Dad's hugs were the best.

As I squeezed Dad tightly, I breathed in his scent. He smelt like toothpaste.

Danielle, Brett and Matthew all chimed together, 'Good luck, Kirsty.'

I smiled, even though my head was still pounding.

Mum reversed our family's white Mitsubishi van out of the driveway and I watched from the front seat as Matthew and Brett ran out onto the front lawn. They began pushing each other. This was a game they played all the time. The aim was to push the other person as hard as you could and see who ended up on their bum first.

As Mum pulled the van onto our street, Matthew and Brett both yelled at the top of their lungs: 'Good luck with *gymSPASTICS!*'

'Little buggers,' muttered Mum.

* * *

I was wearing a jaw-aching smile. Strangers crowded around me, shaking my hand and congratulating me. Then a man with huge muscles pushed through the crowd and held my hand between his giant, grown-up ones.

'You did extremely well today and I think it would be a really good idea if you came and trained with me. Would you like to compete in the Olympics?'

All I could do was nod. I couldn't believe it. Not only had I won a gold medal, but the man that we all knew trained girls who went to the Olympics was telling *me* I could be an Olympic gymnast.

'Here's my card. Tell your mum or dad to give me a call next week to have a chat, okay?'

'Okay, thank you.'

This is the best day ever!

Brett and Matthew didn't congratulate me for winning

when I got home, but they were very happy when they found out we were having Chinese for dinner. We even got to have honey prawns.

All through dinner, whacks of pain smacked my brain. My headache hadn't let up all day and now I had pins and needles in my hands and feet. I had no appetite and could only manage a few mouthfuls of fried rice and a spring roll, even though I hadn't eaten at the competition at all. Mum had been cranky with me because I wouldn't eat the Vegemite sandwiches and apple that she'd brought along for me.

'Are you going to eat a bit more?' asked Mum, with a worried frown appearing between her eyebrows.

'Sorry, Mum. I don't feel hungry. I'm really tired and I just want to go to bed.'

'Bed?!' exclaimed Brett. 'It's only 6.30, who goes to bed that early? You're a weirdo.'

'Brett—' cautioned Dad.

Brett shut up straight away.

'Before you go to bed, your father and I have something we want to give you,' said Mum.

I was surprised. We usually only got presents on our birthdays and at Christmas. Dad held out a small white box.

'What's this for?' I asked.

'Well, you've been working very hard lately at training and we thought we'd get you something to let you know we're proud of you,' explained Dad.

I opened the box and inside was a delicate silver locket. It was heart-shaped with tiny flowers engraved on it, and there was an empty space inside for a photo. I had always wanted a locket.

'Hopefully you'll keep the locket until you're all grown up and you can put a photo of somebody special in there.' Dad lifted the locket out of the box and put it around my neck.

A gold medal, a locket and an Olympic dream coming true all in one day.

I put the trainer's business card under my pillow and went to bed wearing the locket and the medal. Even though my head felt like there was an animal inside it, scratching at my brains, I felt like a champion.

CHAPTER 3

Diagnonsense

I had the biggest crush on a boy called Amos, who was new to my Grade 4 class with Mr F. On his first day at our school he did a dance to a song by Vanilla Ice for our whole class. He had blond hair, blue eyes, and a tiny yellow stud in his left ear. He was really good at drawing and I would stare at his hands when it was art time. I was mesmerised by the fact that he could just look at any object or person and then make them appear in pencil on a piece of paper. He could draw with both his left and right hand. I'd never known anyone who could do that. One day I tried putting a pencil in my left hand and writing my name and it was a squiggly mess. How did he do it?

Amos, of course, had no idea I liked him. You don't tell *anyone* when you have a crush in primary school and you need to act like you hate the boy who you'd actually like to kiss.

On Monday, I wore the gold medal I'd won on the weekend and my new silver locket to school. I was feeling very shiny on the inside as I went into the bag room to get my colouring pencils, and was happy to find Amos there, even if he wasn't alone. My classmate Kate was there too. But as I unzipped my backpack, I felt the hairs on my forearms begin to tingle. Something was wrong.

'You're a fat pig!' he yelled at Kate.

Kate started crying. I was devastated to hear such wickedness gushing from his mouth.

'Leave her alone!' I shouted.

Amos grabbed my shoulders. With his fingers digging into my skin, he shoved me backwards into a cupboard. My head flung back and cracked into the wood. I had never hit my head so hard. My brothers grabbed, pushed and punched me all the time, but it never *really* hurt. Amos had *really* hurt me.

The bag room disappeared. Things went from black to dark purple, and then I could see again. My ears were ringing. Amos pressed his forehead into mine. I could feel a lump swelling to life on the back of my head. He had me pinned up against the cupboard like he was a giant and I was a puny beetle. His blue eyes looked watery.

Why does he look like he's about to cry when he's the one being so mean?

He let me go and stumbled backwards, using his fists to wipe his tears away before us girls could spot them. I rubbed the back of my head. There was no blood, but I had an egg-shaped bump. I watched Amos walk away, his footsteps clunking as he left the bag room. He looked like he was walking wonky, but my eyes weren't working right. I squeezed them shut and opened them again, and the world stopped wobbling.

Kate sniffled. 'Are you okay?'

'Yeah ...' I said. 'We should tell Mr F.'

'No way!' she said. 'Amos will call us dobbers.'

I knew Kate was right. We went back into the classroom and sat down. Amos kept staring at me from across the group of desks for what seemed like forever. We'd made the right choice deciding not to dob on him.

* * *

My home was a very short walk from school, but today the distance was an elongated tunnel. I still had a lump on my head. My eyes felt like they were too big for their sockets. Each step felt like my shoes were made of bricks. There were now even more bruises on me than there had been yesterday.

About twenty metres from home, I got the urge to vomit. Clumsily, I tried to run, but my body wasn't behaving the way my brain was asking it to. My school bag was pulling me down. Air wasn't getting into my lungs. My bones were ice, but my skin was fire.

What's wrong with me?

I managed to make it home and to the bathroom, yanked the toilet seat up and violently threw up into the blue water. On my knees, bent over the toilet, I spewed and spewed. Soon, there was no vomit left, so I heaved up empty mouthfuls of agony instead. I clutched at my cramping tummy with both hands. Tears and snot were oozing down my face. Liquid from my belly had splashed up into my hair. There hadn't been time to pull it out of the way.

I slumped onto my bum next to the toilet bowl and tried to call out to Mum, but it was like being in a dream where you try to scream and nothing comes out. I tried again. This time, I managed to make a sound, but I wasn't loud enough. With my head erupting in pain, and my hands gripping my stomach, I used the only teaspoon of strength I had left.

'MUM!'

Boom! Boom! Boom! Mum's footsteps got closer, as I heard her making her way from the laundry. She appeared in the doorway.

'What's wrong? You look terrible. Why did you walk home from school? I could've come and picked you up.'

'My tummy *really* hurts. I've had a headache for a few days now and it just won't go away.'

Mum quickly grabbed a facecloth, blasted it with cold water and pressed it against my face. 'How bad is the tummy pain? What's it feel like?'

'It feels like someone is stabbing me in the guts.'

She looked at my face and again she stared at the bruises on my legs. 'I think we better go to the hospital. Your appendix might need to get cut out.'

My appendix! This is pretty serious.

I knew what the appendix was and that some people had to have emergency surgery to get rid of it. But I wasn't scared. I just wanted to feel better.

I need to be healthy so I can start training for the Olympics.

* * *

Dad carried me into the emergency waiting room at Sutherland Hospital. My gold medal–winning legs had stopped working and I couldn't keep my eyes open for longer than a few moments. I could feel Dad carefully place me in a hard plastic chair. Then I heard one of the nurses come over.

'How long has her skin looked so yellow and bruised?' she asked.

'She's a gymnast, so she has bruises a lot of the time, but over the last few weeks she seems to have got more,' I heard Mum explain. I felt her warm hands and then the cold hands of the nurse lifting my arms and legs for closer inspection.

'And the yellowness? How long has she looked yellow like this?'

'I don't know,' Mum answered. 'I didn't notice it until now, under the lights in here. What does it mean? Is it serious?'

'I think you should take her to Prince of Wales Children's Hospital in Randwick. Let me go and find the registrar.'

I heard her footsteps disappearing and felt Dad's arm around my shoulders, as he tried to hold my body up in the chair.

Then I heard a man's voice say, 'What's her name?'

'Kirsty,' said Mum.

I felt another set of hands gently lifting my arms and legs for inspection.

'I agree you should take Kirsty to Prince of Wales. You can drive her or we can get an ambulance to take her.'

'We'll drive her,' said Dad. 'Is there any particular reason you can't admit her here?'

'We could take her through and run some tests, but the hospital in Randwick is a specialist children's hospital and I think they'll be better equipped to find out what's going on with your daughter. I'll call them and let them know you're on the way.'

Dad scooped me up into his arms and carried me to the van. He lay me down on the back seat and put the seatbelt around my middle. I felt like the world was made up of fuzzy cotton wool, though there was an occasional blast upon my senses. Even our family van, usually noisy with gear changes, was quiet all the way to Randwick. Then Dad was carrying me again and I heard a barrage of voices of strangers who all sounded like they were hurrying.

'Take her straight through.'

'Get the gas ready.'

'We need to take bloods and do an LP and BMA.'

'Give her a general anaesthetic. She doesn't need to be awake for this.'

What are they talking about?

Dad's arms placed me on a hard bed on my side.

'Kirsty, take some long deep breaths for us.' A rubber mask was placed over my mouth and nose. Sticky, sweet and salty air crawled out of the mask and into my body. The special air made me feel like I was floating away.

'Get the parents to wait outside. They don't need to see this,' I heard someone say and then everything went dark purple.

* * *

I awoke in a hospital bed. A needle was stuck into and taped to the back of my hand. A long tube of blood attached to the needle went up to a bag of blood that was hanging on the top of a metal pole. My lower back and right hip had a sort of stinging and aching pain pulsating inside them.

What did they do to me when I was asleep? I sort of feel better, but my body feels like it has dry ginger ale bubbling and fizzing inside it. They'll probably let me go home soon and then I can get back to school and gymnastics.

My parents came into the room. They looked odd and seemed jumpy.

It's probably the tube stuck into me that's bothering them.

'We're just going to go for a walk up to the end of the ward. Some people want to talk to you,' said Mum.

A nurse unplugged my transfusion pole and helped me out of bed.

I can move my legs! They must've made me better when they put me to sleep.

The nurse pushed the pole while I walked along beside it.

The room at the end of the ward was filled with old brown couches that you could open up and turn into beds. It had a yucky smell, a mixture of smelly feet and armpits with Glen 20 sprayed on top. They sat me down on one of the icky couches, and Mum and Dad sat down next to me. The fabric felt itchy on the backs of my legs.

I don't like this ugly stinky room.

There were a lot of people in the room and they were all strangers to me. My eyes latched on to the oldest person in the room. He was wearing a suit and tie like Dad did every day he went to work, but this man was also wearing a vest under his jacket and there was a watch on a chain pinned to the pocket of his vest. He had a kind face and wore half-moon glasses and I also noticed he had a twitch in his right eye.

Why does this old man look nervous?

Then the old man spoke. 'Hello, Kirsty. I'm Professor Darcy O'Gorman-Hughes. How are you feeling this morning?'

I shrugged. 'I'm okay. Can I go home soon?'

All the adults began looking at each other, except Mum and Dad, who kept their eyes on me.

'Yes,' said the professor. 'You'll be able to go home soon, but you're going to have to come back. You're very sick. You have leukaemia, which is cancer of the blood. That's why you've been feeling nauseous and dizzy, and getting headaches and bruises. The bruises you've had on you are called petechiae. That's just a strange name for bruises that are shaped like circles. They can mean there is something wrong with your blood.'

My whole body felt prickly, like ants were biting my skin. I had never heard of this leukaemia thing, but I'd heard of cancer. My uncle Ken had died of cancer. I remember one day I was sitting on his lap and laughing because he was telling the funniest jokes. He didn't even look sick. He died a few days later. If he died of cancer, that must've meant I was going to die too.

I'm only nine years old. I can't die yet! That's not right.

I felt tears well up in my eyes and I put my hands over my face. I didn't like crying in front of all these people.

'*Don't cry*,' said Mum.

'You're going to be okay,' said Dad.

I don't think parents are allowed to lie to their own kids, so if Dad is saying I'll be okay, then I just have to believe him. Dad wouldn't sit here and lie to me — would he?

The professor began to speak again. 'We're going to give you special medicine called chemotherapy to help you get better. Some of the medicine will be tablets and some of the medicine will be needles. Lots of people your age get leukaemia and with treatment they get better. Most patients who have the same cancer as you have about a seventy per cent chance of getting better. Now, some of the medicine we're going to give you is going to make you feel sick and tired, and give you aches and pains, and with some patients their hair falls out.'

What? My hair is going to fall out and I'm going to have needles and tablets and feel sick?

'Am I still allowed to do gymnastics?' I knew what the answer was going to be, but I had to hear it from him.

'Probably not. You won't feel like doing much anyway.'

It felt like there were spiders inside my throat that were all trying to make webs at the same time, but there wasn't enough room.

Through the spider festival, I choked out another question. 'Can I still go to school?'

'You can go to school if you feel well enough. It's up to you. Some cancer patients take a break from school, or do home schooling—'

'I want to go to school,' I burst out.

'We need to concentrate on making sure you get better. The chemotherapy will help put you into what's called remission. You see, there isn't a cure for cancer, but we do have treatment that we know has worked for other people and we have every reason to believe it's going to work for you. You'll need to be on treatment for about two years.'

Two years?

I felt like I'd been kicked in the stomach.

No gymnastics for two years. No school. No Olympics.

I didn't know what to say to any of the people in the room. I wanted to sit on this ugly brown couch and cry, but Mum had told me not to.

This isn't right. Why is this happening? What did I do wrong?

As if reading my thoughts, the professor continued, 'We don't know why people get cancer and it's not contagious. Some people are just unlucky, but maybe one day, with lots of research, we'll be able to figure out why people get it and then we can find a cure for it. But for now, the best way to get you better is to treat you with chemotherapy, so that's what we're going to do.'

Chubby tears escaped from my face. I tried to hold them in, but they were too heavy for my eyes.

'Don't cry,' said Mum again.

I carefully looked at both Mum and Dad. Their eyes were wild, as though something had startled them. They had the same look as Mum did the time there was a blue-tongue lizard in our backyard, only this time their eyes were even wider. Mum's eyes were swollen. Dad's were still aqua blue, but the white parts looked like a cat had scratched at them. They both blinked a lot. They both seemed to be sitting very still. They both looked like stunned robots who could only open and shut their eyelids repeatedly and not do anything else.

Mum and Dad have both been crying! This must be really bad. I've never seen my parents cry. They've been crying because of me. I've made them sad because I'm sick. They both look so worried and tired, and it's my fault.

'We're all going to help you get better, all right?' said Dad.

'All right,' I said. Dad was the smartest man I knew. I looked around at all the strange people in the room and gave them a half-charged smile. 'So my treatment will be about two years? Does that mean I'll be in hospital for two years?'

'No,' said the professor. 'There will be times where you may have to stay for a few days to have treatment, but we'll try to make sure you spend as little time in here as possible.'

Thank goodness!

'And my hair, you said it might fall out?'

'Yes.'

More tears wanted to push their way down my cheeks. I looked at Mum.

'Don't cry,' she said.

So I didn't.

CHAPTER 4

Kid Are Always Listening

I lay in the hospital bed underneath the stiff white sterile bedsheets. Healthy blood was being poured into my veins through an intravenous line. That's the thing with cancer of the blood — leukaemia — your body needs to be constantly filled with the blood of strangers. I had an insatiable thirst for that scarlet fuel and, without it, I knew I would die.

There was a girl in the bed opposite mine. I didn't know her name, but lots of people came to have whispered conversations around her bed. I heard all of these. I didn't want to and I wasn't trying to, but just like there are some things in life that we can't unsee, there are also things that we can't unhear.

That day, it was the girl's parents and a middle-aged woman wearing a grey business jacket and matching grey skirt. I saw this woman point at me and in a hushed voice she said: 'That little girl has exactly the same cancer as your daughter and we're already working towards getting her better. She has a *seventy per cent chance* of surviving.'

At least I hadn't heard her whisper, 'That little girl over there is going to die.'

She was speaking to the parents, and the girl zoomed her eyes back and forth between them. Left. Right. Left. Right. From father to mother and back. Both parents had their arms firmly folded across their chests. They didn't look at their daughter, at the woman or across at me. I waited to hear their response. Surely *someone* was going to say something.

Why are they all just standing there?

Then, simultaneously, with their gazes glued upon one another, the parents shook their heads.

'No'? What do they mean 'no'? What are they saying 'no' to?

The woman sighed heavily and said softly, 'Okay then. I think someone has already explained what will happen if this is your decision.'

The three adults left the room, their faces looking as if an invisible force was pulling them down to the floor. The girl rolled onto her side and lifted her knees up to her chin. We were totally alone in the room.

'Hey!' I called out to her.

She rolled onto her back.

I know she can hear me. Why won't she answer?

I tried again: 'HEY!' I was loud this time so she couldn't ignore me.

'Ssshhh!' she whispered. 'I'll get in trouble if I talk to anyone.'

'How old are you?'

'Seven,' she said.

She's younger than me?! That's not right. Seven is way too young to have cancer. I'm nine. Nine, I think, is maybe okay, but not younger than nine.

She turned back onto her side again. Our conversation was over, but I wanted to ask her more questions. Maybe I could ask her tomorrow.

I lay there for several minutes staring up at the glaring lights that stung my eyeballs. I found fatigue forcing me to sleep. Cancer makes you feel tired. It's a tiredness that demands to be surrendered to. You just can't fight it, even though hospital beds are impossible to feel comfortable in. The sheets are cleaned and starched so hard that it's like lying between big sheets of paper. The mattresses have plastic covers on them that you can feel through the thin sheets. I guess they were covered in plastic for practical reasons. I couldn't even begin to imagine what bodily fluids had been on this bed before I was in it. Another awful thing about sleeping in hospital beds is how hard it is to find a comfortable position to lie in without accidently ripping out your intravenous line or any other tubes that have been attached to your body. The pillows are also hard, and the plastic oxygen prongs up your nose make your nostrils dry and your snot rock solid. Then there is that horrid smell that lives inside all hospitals.

I went to sleep despite my discomfort, and when I woke up later it was night-time. I knew that, because at a certain time the hospital was kind enough to turn off *some* of the blasting bright lights. I suppose this was to help us sleep, but it didn't help me much because every thirty minutes a nurse would come in to take my temperature and check my pulse. I never slept through a nurse's round. Most nurses didn't seem to care whether you were sleeping or not and would turn on the lights and fumble around your bed. Sometimes there were nice nurses, though, who crept in and used a torch and actually attempted to not wake you up.

On this particular night, I had a nice nurse. If I'd opened my eyes, she would have had a chat with me, but I didn't. She gently took my pulse and temperature, and fiddled with my IV. Her hands were cool and soft.

After she had left, I sat up to see if the girl was awake. I wanted to try to talk to her again.

Her bed was empty and had been made up as if she had never been there.

The nice nurse returned with another nurse, and I pretended to be asleep again. Then I heard something I wish I could have unheard.

'I can't believe those parents,' whispered the other nurse. 'They've pretty much killed their daughter.'

'I know,' the nice nurse replied. 'They wouldn't let us give her a blood transfusion when she first came in. I mean, I understand people having religious beliefs to make life go down a bit easier, but without treatment that kid is gonna be dead in less than two weeks, I reckon.' Then the nice nurse said exactly what I was thinking: 'It's so sad.'

'Well,' said the other nurse, 'kids don't get to pick their parents.'

'It's just so wrong,' said the nice nurse. 'That poor little girl. I wonder what's going through her mind right now?'

CHAPTER 5

The Creature in the Mirror

I still get a surge of delight any time I arrive home, but there's one homecoming I'll never forget. It was when I first learned what we're all told, but don't often fully appreciate: the simple pleasures in life are indeed where we can find the greatest joy.

My homecoming wasn't a comfortable one. Several weeks had slipped by since being diagnosed with cancer and beginning treatment. On the drive home, I had a fiery rash all over my body. Chemicals now lived in my blood. My head felt as if prickly-legged insects were crawling on it, but I didn't dare to scratch. My hair was finding it hard to cling to my scalp. I was afraid that if I touched it, it would slip off, leaving me bald. I wasn't ready for this to happen yet.

Mum pulled the van into the driveway. The crunching sound of the gravel underneath the tires invoked a joyful rush of adrenaline in every cell of my body. In the front yard stood Danielle, Brett, Matt and our family friend and neighbour Linda. As I got out of the van, Linda came rushing up to me and hugged me.

This is weird. Linda has never hugged me before. Cancer must make some people hug you.

Linda hugged Mum too, which was even stranger, as Mum wasn't one for hugging anybody.

Danielle, Linda and Matt ushered me into the house and steered me towards my bedroom. The door was shut, which filled me with panic. Mum had many rules in our home growing up. One of them was if you were naughty, you'd get a smack with her wooden spoon. Another rule was that no doors in the house were to ever be shut, except the bathroom door. Not a single door inside the house had a lock on it.

Why is my door shut? Is this still my room? Maybe it's not my room any more because I have cancer ...

Danielle flung my door open and an avalanche of coloured balloons flooded around me.

'Do you like them?' asked Matt, as he kicked a blue balloon high into the air. 'We spent ages blowing them up for you.'

'I love them,' I answered. 'Thank you.'

'Dad will be home soon and he said we can order as much Chinese food as you like.'

Just as he said that, I heard the front door open and Dad's leather shoes glide lightly along the floor. I heard Dad put his briefcase down in the spot in the hallway where he always placed it. He was an accountant for a very big company and wore a suit to work every day. He usually got changed into shorts and a t-shirt as soon as he got home, but today he came straight to my room and gave me a hug.

'It's good to have you back,' he whispered.

After weeks of barely eating anything in hospital and having just begun a high dose of steroids, which had really increased my appetite, that first dinner back at home was a dance of euphoria upon my tongue and teeth. The honey prawns ... oh, the sickly sweet, deep-fried, sesame-covered honey prawns were the most incredible thing I'd ever eaten. My heightened sense of taste and smell made the flavours explode in my mouth.

And it wasn't just the food. My bedroom, Dad's hugs, even Brett and Matt bickering over who got the last spring roll — these simple things gave me the sensation you get when you're listening to your favourite song: beautiful, perfect pleasure.

That night my bed was a cloud of comfort. It felt so wonderfully strange to not be connected to any tubes. When I needed to pee, I could walk myself to the bathroom instead of having to buzz a nurse and get into an argument, because nurses always wanted me to pee in a bedpan and I always insisted they help me wheel my drip to the bathroom.

I reached under my pillow. The trainer's business card — my golden ticket to the Olympics — was where I'd left it.

I pulled it out, tore it up into six pieces, and threw the pieces into my pink bin near the desk on which my many trophies and books sat. I had to destroy it because it would make me cry, and Mum had told me not to cry.

* * *

Days dawdled by. More and more insects with sticky and prickly legs gathered upon my scalp, but I still didn't dare touch it. My hair changed in texture and colour. It no longer shone or looked like golden syrup. It felt and looked like straw and it had begun to clump into insanely tangled birds' nests.

One day, Mum said, 'I think we need to do something about your hair.'

No! No way!

'Come and sit in the lounge room.'

I did as Mum said. With a hairbrush in one hand and a green bucket in the other, Mum sat on the brown couch and I sat on the floor in front of her. We used to sit like this all the time so she could braid my hair, but there would be no braids today; there would be no braids for a very long time.

Brett kneeled on my left and Matt sat cross-legged on my right. Mum placed the bucket behind me and had barely touched the brush to my head before strands of hair started flittering into the bucket. It didn't hurt. Matt and Brett stared unblinkingly at my head, and then Brett got up and left the room. I sat still and remembered what Mum had told me at the hospital: 'Don't cry.'

I just won't look in the mirror. Then I won't know how bad I look.

In less than two minutes, Mum had exterminated the bugs that had been living on my head and filled the bucket with my hair. Matt looked like he was staring at someone he didn't know. We were all without words. Mum bundled my hair into a plastic bag and hid the bag in our linen cupboard behind the towels.

* * *

Danielle, in anticipation of my hair loss, had used her own money to get me a brand-new baseball cap. It was a royal purple–blue colour and had 'Billabong' written across it — the brand that cool kids wore.

'I'm not sure I like it,' I said to her.

A look of irritation flashed across her face.

'I mean, I'm not sure if it suits me. Am I cool enough to wear it?'

'Of course you are,' she said. 'It's so your head won't get sunburned and for when we go out in public. It might make people stare less. I don't want people staring at you. If anyone stares at you … I'll kill them. I think it looks good on you, but it's up to you if you wear it, okay?'

'Okay,' I said. 'Thank you for getting it for me.'

* * *

'Mum?' I called from the lounge in front of the television one morning. It was a school day, but I had not been to school for a while. I had to wait until my immunity was strong enough to be around lots of kids. I would be returning to school very soon and I couldn't wait to be back in the classroom. In the meantime, Mr F had been sending home bundles of work, which I would devour before sending Mum to get me more.

I was still becoming acquainted with my new friend cancer and I wasn't yet used to being bald. I had not even looked in a mirror since all my hair had fallen out.

'Yeah, love?' Mum called from the kitchen.

'I'm hungry.'

'Really?' She was astonished. I hadn't been hungry since the evening I came home, which was weeks ago. I'd go through phases where I would gorge myself and then the nausea would come and my appetite would disappear for days at a time.

'Yeah.'

'Well, how about we drive to Gymea shops and I'll buy you whatever you want to eat?'

I nodded enthusiastically.

'What do you feel like?'

'Umm ... I feel like a Vegemite sandwich on white bread,' I said.

'You can have anything,' she encouraged me.

'Okay … I still want a Vegemite sandwich.'

'What else? Hot chips? A sausage roll? Ice cream?'

'All right. I also want salt-and-vinegar chips and a rainbow-flavoured Paddle Pop ice cream.'

'I think we can manage that.'

She didn't want to leave me home alone, so I stayed in the car as Mum went into the shops at Gymea and purchased my feast. She got herself a sausage roll with tomato sauce and a banana-flavoured Paddle Pop.

When we got back home, Mum set up a picnic for us on the carpet in front of the television. She made my Vegemite sandwich and cut it into four small squares. We popped one of our favourite movies into the VCR to watch while we ate — *Grease*, with Olivia Newton-John and John Travolta. We sang along to all the songs in between mouthfuls of food.

Stuffed and exhausted, I crawled towards the lounge, laid down and shut my eyes. I felt Mum put a blanket over me. It had been a good morning. There weren't many of them, but as long as there were some it made me feel like everything would be okay.

* * *

There was a very loud knock at our front door. It was 4.15 pm on a school afternoon. I scurried into the lounge room, very gently shut the door, and pressed my ear against the door to listen, curious to know who this visitor was, but not wanting them to catch sight of me and my baldness. I heard the front door unlock and swing open, and then the voice of a boy.

'I'm here to visit Kirsty.'

'Who are you, sweetheart? Are you in Kirsty's class?'

'Yes,' he responded.

'Well,' said Mum, 'she's very sick and she looks very different to the last time you saw her.'

'I don't care how sick she is or how different she looks. I need to see her.'

'All right,' said Mum. 'Why don't you wait in the dining room and I'll see if I can find her?'

Danielle burst into the lounge room, almost hitting me in the face with the door.

'Oh my god, Kirst,' she gushed. 'There's some boy here from your school asking to see you.'

'What does he look like?'

'He's cute. He's got blond hair, blue eyes and a tiny yellow stud in his left ear.'

Amos! I can't believe he has come to visit me! Maybe he has a crush on me just like I have a crush on him? But then he was so mean to Kate at school and then there's my bald head. I bet he did like me as much as I liked him, but he won't like me now.

'You should put your hat on,' she said.

47

'I'm not going to wear a hat,' I stated.

'Are you sure? He'll probably act weird when he sees you. He's just a boy. He doesn't understand.'

'I know,' I said, then slid between Danielle's body and the door, and stepped out into the dining room, where Amos was seated at the table. This was my first bald-head unveiling to the world outside of my home.

'Hi, Amos,' I said sheepishly. I was so self-conscious about my appearance that it felt like my head had just been blown up to the size of a beach ball.

Amos looked at me like he'd never met me before. He looked at Mum, then Danielle, and then back at Mum again.

'That's not Kirsty.' He was being deadly serious.

'Yeah, it's me,' I assured him as I rubbed my hand over my head. 'We're in Mr F's class together. I just look different with no hair and because I'm sick.'

I didn't need a mirror to know how bad my appearance was. Amos's face told me everything. He looked down into his lap and his whole body sagged into the chair.

Poor Amos. I must be the worst thing you've ever seen before. I'm sorry.

His face was sad as he continued looking down.

Please look up, Amos! Please, please, please just look up at me for a few seconds and I'll try to make it better.

Then, he spoke quietly, directing his words into our carpet, underneath the floorboards, and right down into the miles of dirt under our house. 'I'm *really sorry* you're sick.'

The way he was saying 'sorry' seemed odd. Lots of people had been saying 'sorry' to me in cards and phone calls. 'I'm sorry to hear you're sick' was said and written to me over and over again. Some people couldn't even choke out the word 'cancer'. But there was something different about the way Amos had just said 'sorry'.

'I'm so sorry I pushed you at school that day,' he went on. 'I didn't mean to push you so hard.'

He thinks that he did this! Oh my goodness! Poor Amos!

'Amos, I didn't get sick because you pushed me,' I said.

'But I pushed you real hard and you smacked your head and then you never came back to school ...'

'No one knows why I got cancer. Even the professor looking after me doesn't know why.'

Amos seemed sceptical.

Danielle stepped in. 'Kirsty's got two brothers who push her all the time. You can't give someone cancer by pushing them. She's still the same Kirsty.'

Am I the same Kirsty? By the look on his face, I'd say I'll never be the same Kirsty ever again.

Amos didn't look reassured in the slightest. He stood up, with his head and shoulders still drooping so low I thought they'd fall off his body. He glanced back at me very quickly. He seemed afraid to hold eye contact for too long.

'I hope you feel better soon. Goodbye, Kirsty.'

'See you soon, Amos,' I said, as Mum saw him out. 'Oh my gosh!' I said to Danielle as soon as he'd gone.

'You haven't looked at yourself in the mirror yet, have you?' Danielle asked.

I hesitated. 'No,' I said, and it was my turn to look down.

Danielle grabbed my hand and led me to her bedroom. 'I think you should look in the mirror, Kirst.'

I could feel my heart thundering inside my chest and my skull.

I don't want to look. Why do I need to look?

She steered me towards her mirror. Then she stood behind me and placed both of her hands on my shoulders. I let out an enormous sigh and looked into Danielle's black-framed mirror. I didn't recognise the girl who stared back at me. She was mostly bald, with a few straggly bits of hair still hanging on to her head. She had no eyebrows or eyelashes.

'Can I please stop looking now?'

'Yes,' she said. We sat on her bed, and for a few moments were silent. Then she said, 'I'm scared you're going to die. Are you scared? What's it like to be so sick and be bald and everything?'

'Shit!' I exclaimed and started cackling because I'd just gotten away with swearing. Mum hadn't heard me. I looked at the creature in the mirror again. 'Shit,' I said, louder this time, and I giggled again.

I've never liked mirrors since then.

CHAPTER 6

The Importance of Pricks

The first few months of chemotherapy is when your body gets slammed with drugs. The trick is to kill the cancer, but not kill you.

This is rather tricky. Our blood is made up of white blood cells, red blood cells and platelets, and they each have a job to do. White blood cells protect our body against infectious diseases and are known as the cells of our immune system. In a healthy body, white blood cells will prevent you from getting the flu when someone sneezes on you. Red blood cells carry oxygen around our body and carbon dioxide to our lungs so it can be exhaled. Platelets are the blood cells that help your body form clots to stop bleeding. If you bump or cut your knee, for example, a signal is sent to the platelets. The platelets then scamper to the site of the damage and create a bruise or clot, and this helps you heal.

Your platelets also stop your body from bleeding forever if you cut yourself.

Chemo kills cancer — but it also murders the healthy red blood cells and platelets. That's why I often needed blood or platelet transfusions while I was on treatment.

It was a scorching summer's day in 1991 when Mum drove me to the children's hospital in Randwick, which was then called the Prince of Wales Children's Hospital. It was a dungeon and it stank like one too. The walls were brown, the bedheads were brown and even the bedside tables were brown. It reeked of old hospital food trays, dust and antiseptic. I was wearing an old blue Billabong t-shirt that once belonged to Dad. It smelt like him, but this poo-coloured palace would soon eradicate any lingering scent of shaving cream and grass clippings. The building itself seemed to sag and droop, and so did I every time I was there.

I'd been on treatment for a few months now. The treatment I was heading in for would involve a three-day hospital stay. I was having seventy-two hours of intravenous chemo. Mum had to fill out lots of paperwork before we got started because I'd be staying overnight. Plastic hospital identification bracelets were secured on one of my wrists and one of my ankles. Then came one of my least-favourite rituals — a registrar finding a vein. The needle would stay in my body for three days, so they had to make sure they got it in me just right. Eventually, in the back of my right hand, she found a vein. As the cannula crawled under my flesh, I wiggled my toes and tried to remember to not hold my breath. I found if I held my breath, anything they did to me would hurt even more. A nurse proceeded to use *a lot* of tape to hold the cannula firmly in place. She then placed a plastic board under my wrist and wound a bandage around my forearm. Around and around went the cream-coloured fabric, until my arm looked like an Egyptian mummy's.

'Try not to move your fingers at all on your right hand,' she said. 'If the needle slips out, we'll have to stop chemo, find another vein and then get the chemo going again and you'll be stuck in here longer than three days.'

Attached to the cannula was a clear tube — a long worm of transparent rubber that climbed all the way up to a rectangular bag that hung on a metal pole and was labelled:

X — POISON — X
WARNING: TOXIC

This was the fluid that would be flooding my body for the next few days.

Also attached to the pole was a blue box with electric red numbers on it. This box controlled the pace of the poisoning. *Beep! Beep! Beep!* The nurse pressed some buttons, and my hand suddenly felt like someone had placed an ice-pack on it. The ice-pack got bigger and bigger as it went all the way up my arm and into my chest.

I had seventy-two hours to get through and only ten minutes had passed.

Mr F had lent me the books *Matilda* and *The Witches*, both written by Roald Dahl. I was about to decide which one to read when ... 'Mum, I have to wee. Am I allowed to go to the toilet?'

'I don't know, love. I'll go and get someone.'

'Hurry.' I felt like I was about to wet my pants.

Mum returned with a nurse, who was holding a plastic bedpan.

'Here you go, Kirsty,' said the nurse in a sing-song voice, as she plonked the plastic piss pot onto the end of my bed and whooshed the curtain around to give me some privacy. 'You'll need to go to the toilet about every ten to thirty minutes over the next few days. It's the way this drug works its way through your body.'

'Every ten minutes?' exclaimed Mum on behalf of both of us.

'Oh, well, not exactly every ten minutes on the dot, but you'll need to expel urine about three to five times per hour. And don't worry if your wee looks a bit green or has a funny smell — it's just the chemo.'

Just the chemo.

Mum and I gave each other a look: *Is she serious?*

There were five other patients in the room — four boys and one girl. They would all hear me pee. The curtain around the bed didn't even go all the way around, so I'd have an audience as well.

No way!

'Am I allowed to walk to the toilet?' I asked.

'Well … yes, you're allowed, but it's just easier to use the bedpan.'

I swung my legs over the edge of the bed and prepared to stand up. The toilet was only a few metres away.

'Most of the other patients use bedpans.'

I inched my bottom off the bed so I was standing.

'Okay,' said the sing-song nurse. 'Whenever you need to go, you need to unplug the drip from the wall. Only use your left hand to push the pole along to the bathroom with you — we don't want you moving that right hand at all. When you come back, plug the drip back into the wall. The battery lasts about thirty minutes, so if you walk anywhere else, keep an eye on the time. If it's not plugged back in after half an hour, it will start beeping. Are you sure you just don't want to use the bedpan?'

'I'm sure.'

I pulled the plug out of the wall. Mum pushed the pole towards the bathroom for me and stopped in the doorway.

'Do you want me to come in there with you?' she asked.

'Nah, Mum. I can do it on my own.'

'All right, I'm going to stand right outside the door. Call out if you need me.'

I nodded and pushed the rattling wheels of the drip along the grey tiles. I heard the door click shut behind me. I scurried to the toilet and yanked my knickers down with my left hand. I lifted my shirt and fell desperately, bum-first, onto the toilet seat. Wee oozed out of me straight away and my body slumped in relief. It was odd to wipe with my left hand, but I managed. I couldn't resist seeing what colour my wee was. That nurse was telling the truth. I giggled at the sight of my bright-green chemo pee.

* * *

No sleep and green pee for seventy-two hours … every week for twelve weeks. Every two weeks, a lumbar puncture. Every day — thirty tablets. Every day — vomit. Every day — aches in my skeleton.

I've heard many people use the phrase 'cancer sucks'. I don't believe this is accurate enough.

* * *

Today was a pin-prick day. That meant that a nurse would prick my finger — 'pin pricks' they called them — and squeeze out droplets of blood into a tiny plastic tube. Then the Prof (as Professor Darcy O'Gorman-Hughes was affectionately referred to) would take a single drop of blood from that tube and put it on a small rectangular piece of glass and look at it under a microscope.

My blood mustn't have liked the pin-prick nurse, because it usually didn't want to come out and see her. I can't say I blame it. Why would it want to come out into the stinking, stupid hospital?

Today was no exception. The nurse collected my forearm under her armpit, and forcefully pressed and wrenched my finger. It felt as if she'd twisted it so hard that she'd disconnected it from my body entirely.

'Come on, I need more than this.' My finger must've still been attached because she was talking to it. We hadn't even filled an eighth of a tube yet. 'Argh!' She gave up and let go. She handed me a cotton ball to press onto my finger. 'I think we'll need to access a vein, but Kirsty's veins are impossible.' This was said not to my finger but to the Prof, who was sitting and waiting with his friend the microscope.

'Oh, I don't believe that anything about Kirsty is impossible,' he said. 'Do you mind if I have a try?' he asked me.

I nodded.

He put a tourniquet on my right arm and handed me a squash ball. I knew it was a squash ball because Dad played squash. 'Squeeze this in your hand for me.'

The Prof began tapping on my right arm, encouraging the vein to come close to the surface of my skin. 'Now, here's a nice juicy one,' he said, as his warm fingers bounced on a vein that had happily come to the surface for him. He wiped the blue bulge with a white square of nose-crinkling antiseptic. He pushed a teensy metal needle, which looked like a butterfly because it had blue flaps on each side of it, into my flesh and, immediately, dark blood oozed into a thin tube. My whole body drooped in relief. It always did once I knew a vein had been safely conquered.

The Prof got what he needed and pulled out the butterfly. He handed me a cotton ball. 'Press hard so you don't get a bruise.' He went back to his microscope and delicately placed a drop of my blood on a glass slide. He peered into the microscope. 'When would you like to make it back to school?'

'Today. I hate missing it and it's school photos today.'

He looked up and smiled. 'Well, in that case we'd better stick a Band-Aid on you so you can get going.'

'Really?'

'Really,' he said and he began scribbling with a pen. He rolled his chair towards me and stuck a Band-Aid on my arm. He'd drawn a smiling pig on it.

* * *

Wigs, when you're bald, are disgusting and itchy things. I didn't wear a wig. I wore cap hats, but only so I didn't get sunburned. Mum had got me the coolest hat ever. It had rainbow-coloured sparkles all over it. I decided to wear it to school for the photos.

But Mrs Mack, one of the teachers, didn't seem to like

twinkly things. 'Oh Kirsty, take off that ridiculous-looking hat! We all know you have cancer.'

I yanked it off my head and tears began to push out of my eyes, but I could push back harder.

'Oh, all right then,' she said. 'If you're going to make a fuss and act like a child, then just wear your silly hat. But you should really be wearing the school hat. Sparkly hats are not part of the uniform.'

I didn't wear the hat for my Grade 4 photo, but I kept my Band-Aid with the Prof's smiling pig on it. The next day, I wore the school hat.

* * *

At recess and lunchtime, I always looked for Melissa in the playground. Melissa was a few years younger than me and she had neuroblastoma. She got cancer when she was two years old.

I was looking for her wig. It was blonde and shoulder-length and sat lopsided on her head. But my eyes could only spot healthy, non-cancer kids.

I went to the girls' toilets to see if she was in there. The smell of urine crushed against my face. Somebody poked me in my back and giggled. It was Melissa.

'The cap came off my central line and I can't get it back on,' she said. She had a permanent intravenous line that had been surgically put inside her body. They're very uncomfortable, but if you have a lot of chemo your veins die and you get 'promoted' to a central line. I hadn't been promoted yet, but the way my veins were going, it wouldn't be far away. I was hoping my treatment would finish before my veins let me down. Melissa had been on chemotherapy since she was a toddler, so her veins had collapsed years ago.

'I'll help you,' I said. We walked further into the toilets and stood in front of the row of taps. Melissa was clutching the small cap inside her white hand. 'My fingers are really numb today, but I'll give it a go.'

'My fingers are numb too. It was hard to pick the cap up off the ground,' she said.

I grabbed the end of her line and held it into the light so I could see. Carefully, I pressed the cap against the end of the tube and turned it clockwise. It was like screwing the lid back onto a tube of toothpaste.

'There you go.'

An older girl came into the toilets. 'Oh, Melissa, you're so cute,' she said, and she picked Melissa up and sat her on her hip, like she was a doll.

'Careful!' I exclaimed. 'She has a central line.'

The girl looked at me blankly. She put Melissa down and disappeared into a cubicle.

'It's okay,' Melissa reassured me. 'She didn't hurt me.'

We held hands, two girls with skin as clear as plastic wrap, and walked out into the playground together.

CHAPTER 7

Questions with No Answers

Even though it wasn't Christmas, our family was going to Aunty Pat's house. I loved her house. She had a cute scruffy-looking dog, a trampoline that turned your feet blue and a rocking horse. She was the only person I knew who owned a rocking horse. It was white with a red leather saddle and matching red reins. It seemed precious to her, so I never just hopped on it. I would almost pop with anticipation as I waited to be invited to ride this lifelike creature.

Aunty Pat is my dad's sister. She has short brown hair, wears thick glasses and has three daughters. It was Aunty Pat's husband, Uncle Ken, who had died of cancer before I was diagnosed. Aunty Pat was now married to a man named Brian. Dad also has a brother, who has two daughters with his wife, and then there are his parents — Nana and

Grandad. Now that I had cancer, we seemed to be seeing my grandparents, aunties, uncles and cousins more often, though we mostly only spent time with Dad's family. Mum had two brothers and a sister, but she didn't seem to ever want to visit them. One of her brothers was adopted. As for her other brother, Uncle Les — Mum always said us kids shouldn't believe anything he said because he smoked too many drugs. Her sister, Aunty Sandra, lived by herself in Newcastle with two of my cousins. Mum said her sister didn't have much money and that she had to work all the time because her husband was a bad man who she had had to get away from. Mum's mother had died from a heart attack when Mum was only nineteen years old, and her dad had died of cancer a few weeks after I was diagnosed.

Do all the grown-ups think I'm going to die like Uncle Ken? I don't feel like I'm dying. Wouldn't I feel something? Wouldn't I know? I know I could die, but the Prof told me there's a very good chance I'll get better.

I softly stroked the rocking horse's tail and waited for Aunty Pat to tell me I could get on. Pins and needles from the chemo buzzed in my hands and feet. Aunty Pat gave me the nod. Danielle lifted me up and placed me on the shiny saddle. Gently, I began to whoosh back and forth. I gripped the red reins with my tingly and transparent hands. Needle-hole marks were tattooed all over my hands, wrists and arms. Each hole was surrounded by a circle of blue or purple or yellow bruises.

'Do those doctors think you're a pin-cushion?' asked Aunty Pat.

'They say I'm difficult because my veins are hard to find.'

She scoffed. 'I don't believe you're difficult and you shouldn't believe that either. Maybe *they* need to be better at finding veins.'

I'd never thought of that before.

I kept whooshing back and forth on the horse, looking at my frail fingers. My hands and arms wouldn't be strong enough to hang from the bars at gymnastics any more.

Mum came over. 'Pat,' she said, 'Kirsty's gotta take her tablets.'

Aunty Pat turned to me. 'Can you take them with lemonade?'

Yum! Lemonade instead of my usual orange cordial ...

'Yes, please!'

I sat at the dining table, among the adults and cups of tea on saucers and Scotch Finger biscuits. Aunty Pat got me a whole can of Kirks lemonade, just for me, and poured it into a glass. Mum, having carefully wrapped my thirty or so tablets in plastic wrap before we left home, placed the pile of poison before me.

I stared out longingly at Brett and Matt, who were outside jumping on the trampoline. I was too weak to jump and I knew I'd soon be out of breath if I tried. Brett saw me watching and stuck his middle finger up at me while he leapt into the air. None of the grown-ups saw.

I began taking my tablets, one at a time, one sip at a time. I always waited a few moments in between each tablet to make sure the pill made it all the way down to my belly. If I threw up, I'd have to start all over again.

'Do you remember that day a while back, just before we lost Ken?' said Aunty Pat. 'Do you remember all the attention he was giving to Kirsty? Do you think maybe he knew something that we didn't?'

I'd become used to adults talking about me as if I wasn't there. Even when they acknowledged I was there, they spoke like I didn't understand what they were saying.

'I mean, out of all the kids that day, he didn't seem to want to let Kirsty out of his sight,' she continued.

Tea was slurped and biscuits were crunched. I swallowed another tablet. I liked to swallow the dark-yellow ones first — methotrexate — then the lighter-yellow ones — mercaptopurine — and then I'd swallow the white chunky steroids last.

The thought that my uncle might have sensed something seemed too much for the adults to contemplate and no one offered any response.

Did Uncle Ken know cancer was going to come for me too? Does cancer make you know things other people don't know? I can smell and taste and feel everything so much more now that I've got cancer.

I clasped the locket Mum and Dad had given me in my left hand and picked up the final and most bitter-tasting of all my pills. The steroids — prednisone — were shaped so stupidly. They were like thick flying saucers with sharp ridges instead of smooth ones. I put it on my tongue and took a big gulp of lemonade. The little bugger got stuck so I kept swallowing more lemonade and silently willed it out of my throat and down my body. Eventually the pill obeyed my command, but its sour metallic essence remained in my mouth.

'So,' said Mum, breaking the spell that had been cast around the table, 'are we all ready for Christmas this year?'

Mum was answered with relieved conversations about decorations and wrapping presents and who made the best potato salad. Some things are just too hard for adults to talk about, but there's always Christmas lights and salads.

CHAPTER 8

Sideshow

Westfield Miranda was the place that you went to in the Sutherland Shire when the weather wasn't sunny enough to be at Cronulla Beach. At Westfield, you could go to the movies, get food, look at all the shops, hang out with your friends, or even take your bald head out for an hour or two to see how strangers react. Danielle had offered to take me and Matt, and now she was negotiating the terms and conditions with Brett, who wanted to go to feast on McDonald's and KFC but didn't want to be seen with me.

'I'm not going if Kirsty's going!' Brett fumed. 'Mum!'

Mum's footsteps plodded towards us. 'What's going on? I can hear you all the way out in the laundry.'

'Brett doesn't want to come because he thinks everyone will stare at Kirsty,' said Danielle.

'Everyone *is* going to stare at her. It's embarrassing,' said Brett.

'Brett,' Mum said, flustered and fed up as she often was with us, 'that's not a very nice thing to say. Kirsty can't help being sick.'

'But Kirsty looks like the witch out of *Robin Hood: Prince of Thieves*!'

'Brett!' Mum snapped.

It was true. Just like that witch, I was mostly bald, with little blonde wisps of hair still grasping to my head. You often see people with cancer depicted as having these perfectly smooth bald heads, but mine didn't look like that.

'I'll wear my Billabong hat,' I offered. It wouldn't make any difference to me. With or without a hat, I still had cancer, but if it would make Brett feel better I'd wear it.

We all piled into the family van and Mum drove our noisy Mitsubishi to Westfield. She dropped us off outside the main entrance, near a bus stop where twenty or so people were waiting. I hurried along with Matthew by my side, Danielle a few metres in front and Brett further ahead.

A fierce wind smacked at my bare legs and made my eyes water. Suddenly my cap was whipped off my head and skittered far behind me. Hats don't stay on your head very well when you're bald, because there's nothing for the hat to hold on to.

A collective gasp arose from the people lined up. They weren't expecting to see a little girl who looked like the witch from the movie *Robin Hood: Prince of Thieves*.

'Wait!' I called to Danielle through the thick wind. 'My hat!'

Brett turned around. 'Oh great,' he said sarcastically, 'so much for the hat.'

'Shut up, Brett!' said Danielle.

I managed to snatch up my hat, but now that every stranger standing at that bus stop could see I was bald, it seemed silly to cover my head up, so I clutched my hat in my hands. Then I noticed Matt was holding on to me.

'Come on,' I said to my siblings, 'let's split up and meet back here in two hours.'

'Whatever,' said Brett and he walked off. Matt released his hold and galloped after Brett.

'He's such a dickhead,' said Danielle.

'Hey,' I said, 'I've always wondered … does being a dickhead mean you have a dick attached to your head or that your whole head is actually a dick?'

'I don't know,' she replied.

Danielle and I went to my favourite store. As Brett would say, they sold 'hippy crap'. Among the dream-catchers and incense, a mother and daughter were looking at some necklaces inside a glass display case to my right, while not far away from me to my left, Danielle was looking at a book about talking to the dead. I picked up an orange-scented candle called Citrus Delight and sucked in its sticky sweet smell through my nostrils. With my heightened sense of smell, I was obsessed with smelling things.

As I put the candle back down, I became very aware of the mother's eyes diving into my baldness. Brett was right. People were staring. I tried to ignore her and picked up a lavender candle. I read the label: 'Lavender creates feelings of calmness and relaxation.' I sniffed really hard and loud. It didn't work at all. I didn't feel calm or relaxed. Snubbing the staring woman was harder than I thought.

Please stop staring at me and go away.

I wished the words inside my head and my wish was granted. She started to walk away. I licked my chemo-cracked lips and turned to look at the crystals, but this woman was now standing right in front of me. There was only about a metre between us. She was gripping her daughter's hand. They looked at me like they were at the circus and I was the bearded lady. I pretended that my attention was drawn to the dream-catchers hanging from the ceiling. I tried so hard to fixate on the feathers and beads that dangled over my head.

Then the woman spoke to her daughter. Everybody in the shop could hear her. 'Darling,' she said, not taking her eyes off me for a second, 'look at how strange that little girl is.'

At hospital, when things hurt, they tell you to wiggle your toes. I wiggled my toes. My heart thudded. I didn't cry. I didn't run. I didn't even blink, but I did wonder what Danielle was going to do. She was already striding towards my audience. Still fascinated by me, they didn't notice her approaching.

A lavender candle wasn't going to help Danielle calm down right now. In a strong clear voice, she bellowed, 'One of the most important lessons a mother should teach her daughter is that it's *very rude* to stare.'

The glaring duo stared downwards in shame.

'Let's go,' I said quietly and grabbed Danielle by the hand.

We walked out, Danielle, the lioness, stalking with big strides, and me, the mouse, scurrying to keep up. 'What a *fat* bitch!' she spat out.

'So ...' I said, 'do you think that woman had a dick attached to her head or that her whole head was actually a dick?'

* * *

Apart from the hospital, there weren't many places where I wasn't the strange creature for people to stare at, but cancer camp was one of the places where I didn't feel so excruciatingly like the odd one out. There were over two hundred people at cancer camp. One hundred of those people were kids just like me who had cancer. Each of us was assigned a volunteer, a grown-up to keep a watchful eye over us. There were also nurses and a couple of doctors — all of whom were volunteers — who came along to make sure that we had fun, and, if anything went wrong, they'd take care of us. I didn't really like going, but I thought it would be nice for my family to have a break from me, my baldness, my cancer and all the rubble it brought into their lives.

The best thing about cancer camp was that I got to spend time with Melissa. We got to do all sorts of fun activities together, and this afternoon there was going to be a piggy-back race.

Before the race, Melissa and I decided to go for a dip. There was a huge lake at the camp and to get to the lake you had to cross a huge open field of grass. The only bad thing about this stunning location was that the grass was riddled with bindies. The day we arrived, they warned all of us to never walk barefoot on the grass.

The lake was forever at low tide. You could walk out one hundred metres and the water would only come up to your knees. Melissa and I took our thongs off at the edge of the lake and splashed about in the cool water as we waited for the piggy-back race to start. Melissa wasn't wearing her wig and I wasn't wearing a hat. We didn't need to worry about our bald heads bothering anyone when we went to camp.

Suddenly, our volunteer companions yelled at us to come out of the water. 'Come on, you two! The race is about to start!'

We charged through the water and climbed onto the backs of our adult companions.

'We're going to win!' Melissa teased the other kids and companions, and her eyes sparkled with their own special breed of mischief.

'We'll see about that!' I yelled back at her.

One of the nurses held up her hand to start the race. 'On your mark, get set, GO!'

Off we went, bobbing up and down as we clung on tightly. Delight-filled screams of 'Go faster!', 'Hurry up!' and 'We've gotta come first!' could be heard as the adults did their best to run with sick kids clinging onto their backs like white-skinned monkeys. We charged along the field, getting closer and closer to the finish line.

'Faster!' I heard Melissa squeal and her companion rushed forwards ahead of us to win the race. In gymnastics, second place was unacceptable for me, but in this race, I was glad to be second behind Melissa. 'Wooooooohooooooo!' she yelled, as her companion ran around in victory circles.

My companion set me down on the path at the top of the field and eventually Melissa was set down too. We were given our medals.

'I beat you, I beat you!' Melissa taunted me playfully.

'It's probably 'cause you're smaller than me,' I replied.

Sarcastically she retorted, 'Excuses, excuses ... I'm the winner! Wooohooo!'

'All right, all right. You're the winner.'

She flung her arms around my middle and squeezed.

'Okay,' one of the doctors announced, 'everyone back to their cabins for "horizontal time" before we head out for bowling tonight.' Horizontal time was rest time. Every afternoon the campers were supposed to lie down and have a rest, as we had activities on during the day and night, and we did have cancer.

'Oh no,' I said.

'What's wrong?' asked Melissa.

'Our shoes! Our shoes are down by the lake. We didn't put them back on before the race started.'

She started chuckling. Our companions had already started to walk back to our cabins.

'How are we going to get our shoes?' I said. 'The bindies are everywhere.'

Melissa thought for a moment. 'Let's run,' she said.

'What? No way!'

'If we run as fast as we can and keep going no matter how many bindies we get in our feet ... we can make it.' With her grin, she dared me to run the gauntlet. 'Come on ... don't be chicken.' She began making clucking sounds.

'Okay, okay, I'll do it. As long as I can swear and yell as much as I need to!'

'Of course, just don't stop running no matter what,' she instructed. 'On the count of three. Ready?'

'No,' I whined.

She laughed at my reluctance. 'One, two, THREE!' Barefoot, we bolted as fast as we could along the field that was infested with sharp bindies.

'Ow! Shit!' I exclaimed.

'Don't stop! Keep running!' she yelled, as we both kept up our charge towards the water's edge. 'Ouch!' She stumbled slightly but kept going as we'd promised.

Countless sharp, dry and hard bindies dug themselves deep into the soles of our feet. I started to scrunch my toes together, but that didn't help.

'Crap!' Melissa cried out.

'Keep going!' I urged her. 'We're almost there! Ah, bugger!' I almost fell on my face as more of the painful weeds pierced my skin. 'I'm going to leap on the sand!' I yelled.

'Good idea!' she hollered back at me. As we got closer to the sand near the water's edge, we timed our leap to safety. 'Ready?!'

'Yep! Shit! Yes! Ready!'

'Now!' she called out. We both stretched out our arms and launched our bodies belly-first onto the sand.

We had made it. We were both panting, unaccustomed to running, and then Melissa erupted in giggles. We rolled around on the sand laughing and trying to breathe. Eventually we sat up and began helping each other pluck the merciless bindies from our feet.

'I've never run like that ever in my whole life,' she panted with glee.

Our adult companions couldn't understand why we wouldn't stop giggling during horizontal time.

CHAPTER 9

A Short Walk Home

It only took five minutes — ten if you dragged your feet — to get home from school. One of the things that I adored most about the walk was the gumtrees that lined the entire route. The ghost gums stretched up over me, forming a protective canopy over my head, and the leaves on the ground were my own red carpet. The leaves still on the trees made soothing whooshing sounds that kept me company. It was almost like the trees were speaking to me.

Mum had told Brett to collect Matt from the infants' part of school on Friday and walk him home. She didn't say Brett had to collect me, and even if she had he would've said he forgot. They were already through the school gates and a block or so along the street when I spotted them. I could see Brett's rusty mop of hair bobbing along the footpath and Matt's jet-black spiky hair and his stocky legs as he struggled to keep up with his big brother. The gumtrees over my head weren't speaking to me today.

'Brett! Matt! Wait up!' I yelled.

Matt turned around. He grabbed Brett's arm and pointed at me. Brett yanked his arm free and kept walking. Matt hovered for a few moments, then chased after Brett. Then behind me I heard, 'Get her! Get the freak!'

On the back of my bald head I felt a *thud*, then a long heavy scratchy *bang* smashed into the back of my shoulders. Rocks and sticks were being fired at me. I no longer had the legs of a gymnast. I had legs made of twigs that were very easy to snap, but I ran anyway. My silver locket bounced in front of my face as I tried to run from the group of girls and boys chasing after me.

'We're gonna get you!'

'My mum said you and Melissa are gonna die!'

'My parents told me I don't have to be nice to you like the teachers told us to!'

The back of my head felt sticky, like they'd hammered me with bullets made of treacle. But as the stickiness crept down the collar of my uniform and down the front of my chest, I could see it was *not* treacle. Their rock and branch missiles were making me bleed.

'Help me!' I called out to my brothers.

Matt stood as still as the trunks of the gumtrees.

Brett kept walking.

Tears began streaming from my eyes and snot blocked my nose. I begged my legs to go faster and for a few seconds they did. I gasped for air as more pebbles struck me. The rocks hurt more than the sticks. My twiggy legs would stop working soon. I couldn't win this race. I had two options — fall on my face or stop running.

My attackers were right behind me. I turned around. Just as I was about to open my mouth to swear at them, one of the boys swung his school bag at my head. *Clang!*

For a few seconds, I lost my hearing. I could see girls and boys yelling with twisted faces, but all I could hear was a sharp ringing noise. A drop of blood dribbled lazily down my chin and I could taste wet metal in my mouth. Tears gushed out of my eyes like a tap had been turned on. The street no longer had houses or trees in it. It was made of fuzzy shapes and colours.

'Brett! Help me!'

Matt unfroze and dragged Brett towards me. My tormentors bolted back inside the school gates.

'What do you want?' Brett yelled.

'Those kids up there,' I panted, pointing at them, 'those kids hurt me because I have cancer.'

'I didn't see anything.' Brett turned and strode away so fast that he soon disappeared.

Matt, as soundless as the trees, stayed beside me. My frail legs felt flame-licked. Matt took my school bag off my shoulders and carried it for me. Then I heard it and I felt it — a delicate gust whipping through the branches of the trees. I wasn't alone. I had Matt. I had the trees. They kept us company as we walked the short walk home.

* * *

Dad always got up earlier than any of us. It was 6 am on Saturday, so he had already had his Weet-Bix with milk and read *The Sydney Morning Herald*, and now he was in the backyard doing some garden work.

Quietly, I opened the sliding door. I could see Dad's lithe body crouched at the very back of the yard near the pool. He was pulling out nutgrass. I walked barefoot along the grass, still wet from the morning dew, and sucked in the early morning air. It's the best air to breathe — cold and crisp. It smells more enchanting at 6 am than it does at 10 am.

As I got closer, Dad heard my bare feet squishing on the grass and stood up. He was near the tree with the strange cylinder-shaped pink flowers on it. Birds of all kinds were in love with this tree more than any other tree that Dad had planted around the above-ground pool.

'You're up early,' he said.

'Yeah,' I said flatly.

'How are you feeling?'

'My head's sore,' I said, as I rubbed the wounds from yesterday afternoon.

'I'm sure it is,' he said. 'Want a hug?' With my stick-insect legs, I ran at Dad's waist and squeezed. I breathed in Dad's smell of shaving cream and grass clippings, wondering why he always smelt like grass when he rarely mowed the lawn. He waited for me to let go.

I stopped squeezing and looked down at our bare feet. Dad's feet were giant-sized next to mine. 'Why does Brett hate me?' I asked softly. A magpie warbled from the neighbour's wattle tree.

'Why do you think Brett hates you?' he asked calmly, as he took a few steps towards the tree with the strange flowers, startling the birds playing among the branches.

'He ignores me and doesn't want to be near me. I think he hates me because I have cancer.'

Dad began carefully plucking flowers off the tree.

'I was so scared yesterday when those kids chased me and I tried to run, but I could only run for a little bit and then …'

'Then what?' Dad looked down at me for a moment.

'If my legs were strong like they used to be, I would've outrun those kids, but they're not, so I couldn't.'

Dad now had a huge bunch of flowers in his right hand and he began tapping them gently against his left hand. 'Lots of people run when they're scared. People can also get angry and do ugly things when they're scared.'

'Just tell me why Brett hates me. I don't care about those dumb kids, but I want to know why he's so mean to me.'

'He's scared,' Dad said and he stopped tapping the flowers.

'I was scared too.'

'I can't even imagine how scared you must have been.'

'I was so scared, Dad.' The tears began to gush from my eyes. 'I wish that I could run. I wish that I never got cancer. I wish I was a gymnast again.'

'I think Brett was wishing for those things too. I'm not sure that he knows it, but that's what I think.'

I stared at the enormous bunch of flowers in Dad's strong hand. 'So you don't think Brett hates me?'

'Well, I'm not Brett, so I can't know for sure, but people do weird things when they're scared. They can do and say things that don't make sense.' Dad smiled warmly at me. 'Come here and look at this.' He beckoned me closer. On his hand where he'd tapped the flowers sat tiny droplets of water. He turned his hand upside down, but the droplets didn't fall off. He turned his palm upwards again and reached it towards me. 'Taste one.'

I pulled an 'ick' face.

He licked one of the droplets off his thumb. 'Mmm … You should try everything once.'

I stretched out a finger and wiped up a droplet. It didn't feel like water. It was viscous. I put the drop onto my tongue. An eruption of sweetness burst to life inside my mouth.

'Oh my gosh …'

'Want some more?'

I nodded and took another, and then another.

How does Dad know these flowers have lolly drops inside them? How come Dad always makes me feel better? How come he always knows the answers to everything? I wonder if other dads are as clever as my dad.

'Dad!' Brett called from the back door. 'Can we go for a surf?'

Dad rubbed his hands against his yard shorts. 'Sure!' he said. 'We'll go and see if the waves are any good at Greenhills.'

He walked back inside, carrying the bunch of flowers. He'd put them in a vase for Mum.

I tried to follow Dad into the house, but Brett stood in the doorway, not letting me through. With Dad out of earshot, he said, 'You're not coming. You don't even know how to surf.'

I shrugged and shoved him out of my way and went inside to take my morning mountain of tablets.

CHAPTER 10

It Burns

News spreads quickly in the Sutherland Shire.

'Things aren't looking good for Melissa,' Mum said. 'They've sent her home from hospital to make her comfortable. She's not going to get better. Her mum said she keeps asking to see you, but we've spoken about it and decided it's not a good idea.' Mum was a robot as she spoke.

I stared into the wood grain of the dining room table, perfect straight lines of browns and caramels. Then, among the precise lacquered horizontal lines, I saw a dark spot, an imperfection. What had once been a tree was now a table. I could feel Mum's eyes watching me. The regimented lines became a blur as tears threatened to fall from my face.

Melissa is going to die and I'm never going to see her again.

I went to my room and shut the door, even though I knew it might get me in trouble. I sat on the floor, tucked my knees under my chin and the tears shuddered out of me. I sobbed as quietly as I could because I knew Mum didn't want me to cry. The tears felt like acid and burned my cheeks. My t-shirt was soggy with snot and tears, but I didn't care. I kept waiting for Mum to open the door or at least knock on it, but she never did. She was letting me break one of our house rules. Behind a door I'd never closed before, I became a ball of agony.

The grown-ups had decided that Melissa and I could not see each other one last time. They thought it was for the best. They thought it would be too hard on both of us. They thought they were doing the right thing, but was it the right thing?

I couldn't see Melissa, so I wrote her a letter and covered it in stickers.

Dear Melissa,

I'm so sorry that you're sick. I'm sorry I can't see you. Our mums talked and decided it's not a good idea. I really wish I could come and visit you. Do you remember your birthday party? Do you remember when you cut the cake you touched the knife to the bottom on purpose, so you'd have to kiss the boy you had a crush on? I'd never be brave enough to do that. I've never even kissed a boy. You're the bravest person I've ever known.

Love from your friend,

Kirsty. oxoxo

A few days later, Melissa wrote back:

> *Dear Kirsty,*
> *Thank you for the lovely note and the stickers. I wish I could*
> *see you.*
> *Love Melissa. Oxoxo*

She included a drawing of two little girls playing on a swing
set in a park.

* * *

Death calls always arrive early in the morning. I felt it coming.
It was like an invisible hand was scooping everything out of
my tummy, and then the phone rang. Mum answered and had
a hushed conversation.

After she hung up, she went into the lounge room and
slumped down onto the couch. It looked as though she was
having trouble holding her body upright. She put her hands
over her face. She was still in her nightgown and her hair was
a wild mess, as it always was in the mornings. I knelt at her feet
and rested my head on her knee.

'It's okay, Mum,' I said.

Moments dragged and I sat with Mum, waiting for her to
say the words. With her hands still over her face, she finally
spoke.

'Melissa died early this morning. There's going to be a funeral on Friday. You've never been to a funeral before. Your father and I will be going, but everybody will understand if you don't go.'

'It's up to you to decide,' said Dad from his spot in the doorway. He looked as though he'd seen a ghost.

I've never been to a funeral before. What will people think of me if I go to the funeral and I don't cry? Can I tell people I already used up all my tears when I was alone in my bedroom?

An unseen force began tugging at me, pulling me towards my decision.

* * *

I'd never worn all-black clothes before. Mum had to buy me a black outfit, which included black stockings that made my legs itchy.

The funeral was at a place called Camellia Gardens. It's a beautiful place where people have their wedding photos taken. We followed the winding path through the park and came to a clearing near some purple violets. *Purple and pink are Melissa's favourite colours*, I thought and then … *smack!* Right in front of me was a small white coffin with shiny silver handles.

Melissa is inside that coffin.

Something was flogging me from the inside. Broken shards of glass pierced the inside of my throat. Mum tried to stand in front of me to block the sight of the coffin, but she was too late. A woman came up and hugged me and Mum, and said, 'It's okay. Melissa is with God now.'

I nuzzled into Dad's hip. He held my whole head with one of his hands.

Be brave, I told myself. *Be brave for Mum and Dad.*

I looked over at the coffin again. I imagined it was me inside the coffin and not Melissa.

Why isn't it me in the coffin?

* * *

As soon as I got home, I ripped off my prickly black stockings. Then I went hunting through a box of photographs. I found the one I was looking for, cut out part of it into the shape of a tiny heart and put the photo inside my locket.

Mum and Dad had told me, when they gave me this locket, that one day I could put a photo of someone really special inside it.

Nobody will ever be as special as Melissa.

CHAPTER 11

Pigeon House Mountain

For as long as I could remember, our family went camping every year. We usually went somewhere on the South Coast of New South Wales. We slept in a big orange-and-blue tent. We swam in the ocean. We walked through the bush. We let campfire flames hypnotise us every night.

Even though I had cancer, Mum and Dad made sure we still went on our camping trips. This time, we were staying at the Pebbly Beach campground in the Murramarang National Park. I don't know why it was called Pebbly Beach, because the beach wasn't covered in pebbles, it was covered in sand, like all the beaches I'd ever walked on.

The sunlight is always shiniest at sunrise when we're camping. Maybe it was because the tent was mostly made of orange fabric. Nestled inside my green sleeping bag, I could see droplets of morning dew had fallen on us while we slept.

I could also hear Matt's ogre-like snoring coming from the bunk bed below me. Then I heard the careful whizz of a zipper opening on our tent. Dad was getting Brett up to go surfing. I shut my eyes and pretended to be asleep. I felt Dad kiss my forehead and then he gently whispered, 'Brett, let's go. There should be a good swell this morning.'

I heard the carelessly loud fumbling of Brett wriggling out of his sleeping bag. I heard another whizzing zipper, and Brett tumbling out of the section of the tent that he shared with Danielle. I could smell the charcoal from our campfire the night before. I kept my eyes shut and listened to the kookaburras as they tried to laugh us campers awake. I heard Brett and Dad gathering up their surfboards and the flip-flopping of their thongs as they made their way to the ocean. Mum, Danielle and Matt were all still firmly floating in the land of dreams. The kookaburras seemed to fade and I plummeted back to sleep in my warm tube of feathers and flannelette pyjamas.

I awoke to the smell of instant coffee and Vegemite on toast. I climbed out of my cosy tunnel and joined my family at the fold-out camping table. Mum placed an enormous plastic cup of orange cordial and a disposable foam cup containing my tablets in front of me. I started taking my venomous pills. My family filled their tummies with coffee and pineapple juice and toast. I filled my tummy with what was necessary.

'So, are we all ready to climb Pigeon House Mountain today?' asked Dad. He'd surfed and showered and was keen to take us all on a bushwalk to a place we'd never been before. He was wearing aviator sunglasses and a black–and–red t-shirt we'd given him for Father's Day.

A tablet got stuck in my throat and I guzzled down more cordial. The sun warmed the ground and tiny skinks flitted about as they tried to find the sunniest spots to lie in.

'Why's it called "Pigeon House Mountain"?' asked Matt.

'Well, when Captain Cook first came to Australia, he thought the top of the mountain looked like a dove or a pigeon house, like they had back in London. He just named the mountain after what he thought it looked like.'

'If it's too much for Kirsty, her and I won't walk all the way to the top,' said Mum.

'I can do it, Mum,' I said.

'Wait and see how you feel,' she said. 'If you start to feel sick or get too tired, you need to tell us.'

I nodded a fake promise. I felt sick and tired almost all the time.

The tablets squirmed inside my belly.

Don't you dare throw up today, I silently ordered my body.

* * *

'You'd all better go to the toilet before we start walking,' said Mum, 'otherwise you'll have to go in the bush.'

We'd arrived at the bottom of Pigeon House Mountain. You couldn't see the top. All you could see was a trail that led into the bush and a wooden box that contained what must've been the world's most foul-smelling dunny. One by one, we used what Dad told us was a 'pit toilet'. It was a stinking, seething hole in the ground that people filled with wee and poo. As I shut the door, my tablets upheaved into my mouth. I swallowed them back down. They came back up again. I held my nose and swallowed the mixture of half-fizzled-away tablets and cordial back down into my stomach.

I wonder how deep this hole is?

I looked down into the revolting dark hole. A streak of light cut a line through the cubicle and shone down into the pit. I could see rats crawling around among the human waste. Still holding my nose with one hand, I inched my shorts down and ordered my body to wee, even though I kept thinking a rat would crawl up my bum. I scurried out as soon as I was done.

'What's wrong?' asked Matt, when he saw the look of disgust on my face.

'I looked down the hole of the dunny and there were rats down there!'

'Gross!' he exclaimed.

Brett joined us and whispered, 'I heard that they put dead bodies down there when they don't want people to find them, but sometimes the bodies aren't dead and they try to climb out and they're covered in wee and poo.'

Matt's eyes became enormous orbs of terror.

'Us boys should always be careful when we wee into a pit toilet 'cause someone might reach up and grab our dicks!' Brett cackled.

Matt decided to wee against a tree instead.

There was a sign at the beginning of the trail. Mum and Dad always encouraged us to read the signs on bushwalks and try to remember what we had read once we got home. I read it out loud: 'The Aboriginal name for Pigeon House Mountain is Didthul or Didhol, which means "woman's breast".'

Brett nudged Matt.

'Aboriginal people called it this because this is what the mountain actually looks like — a woman's breast.'

'Oh, I don't think that's true,' scoffed Mum.

I quietly tried to pronounce the Aboriginal name of the mountain: 'Didthul ... Didhol ...' I liked how the letters felt inside my mouth and I kept saying them to myself over and over again as we walked through the bush. Like giants clasping their hands together, the trees formed a ceiling of leaves and branches over us as we climbed. Crunchy gravel scratched underneath our sneakers and soon we had to climb over large rocks that were embedded into the path. For about two hours we puffed and panted and climbed closer to the sky on the extremely rugged pathway.

And then: 'Oh! No way, Peter. I'm not climbing up there and I'm not sure any of you should either. If you fall, you'll break your bloody necks.'

I looked up and saw what had provoked Mum. Long vertical metal ladders had been drilled into rocks that went up and up and up.

'But we're almost at the top!' wailed Brett.

'Well, there's no way I'm going any further,' said Mum, as she folded her arms and plonked herself onto a rock. 'How are you feeling, Kirsty?'

I wanted to throw up and my spine was aching, but I said, 'I'm fine, Mum.' I could feel my bald head twinkling with sweat and my heart pumping so hard I thought it might explode. 'I want to go all the way to the top.'

Dad went over to where Mum was sitting and they spoke softly so we couldn't hear them. Us kids stood waiting and panting. Eventually, some agreement must've been reached, because we were all allowed to climb to the top. Mum would wait for us where she was.

Danielle went first, then Brett, who was too cool to show or admit to any concern about heights. Then up went Matt, and then me, and then Dad. Maybe Dad had promised Mum he'd catch any of us if we fell? With Dad right behind me, I wasn't scared at all.

'I want all of you to go slowly,' instructed Dad. 'It's not a race. One step at a time and don't step up until you've got a good grip with both hands and one foot is firmly in place on the metal.'

So the Everett ants, excluding Mum, went marching one by one all the way to the top of the mountain.

'Wooooooohoooooooo!' Brett called out with his hands cupped around his mouth. 'We're standing on a woman's nipple!' We all laughed as Brett did a victory jig on the rock platform.

'Look at that view,' said Dad, as if he couldn't believe how good it was. 'Look, kids, no matter which direction you face all you can see is sky and the tops of the trees.' He faced one way and then turned and faced another, as if he was checking that what he'd said was indeed true.

I copied him. It was true. I didn't feel like throwing up any more and the ache in my back had vanished.

'Look! I'm jumping on a boob!' Brett squealed, as he began jumping up and down. Matt joined in.

Danielle shielded her eyes from the sunlight and gazed all around. 'Wow ... I can't believe Mum is missing out on all of this.'

'She's all right,' said Dad. 'She's afraid of heights.'

While Brett and Matt enjoyed bouncing around, Dad took photos. He loved taking photos. I remember one time Mum got mad at him because he used up a whole roll of film taking photographs of the ocean. She said it was a waste of film. Dad said that every photo was different because the sun had been setting and the colours kept changing. I looked at the twenty-four photos and Dad, as always, was right.

It was time to leave Didthul and climb back down to Mum. In a sing-song voice, Brett chanted as we made our way back to the beginning of the trail: 'I walked on a tit today! I jumped on a giant nipple!'

'All right, Brett,' cautioned Dad, 'I think that's enough about tits and nipples for today,' and we all cracked up laughing. Even Mum couldn't help but smile as we left Didthul.

CHAPTER 12

Methotrexate Murderer

One of the things that used to worry me the most about chemo was that you never knew which registrar you would get. How many times would it take them to get your lumbar puncture right? How many times would it take them to find a vein? How many times would I have to suffer? The Prof was an amazing man, but he was not the one who gave me chemo.

I'll never forget the worst registrar of them all.

I sat on the treatment bed and held out my arm ready for the stranger with smudged glasses and dirty fingernails to start looking for a vein, but he wasn't ready. He didn't speak to me or even look at me. He was standing at the bench opposite with his back to me. On the bench, I could see the manila folder containing my medical file and the small glass phial of methotrexate — the drug I was having injected today. My body had been drowned in oceans of methotrexate.

'Can you give me your Medicare card?' he asked, finally turning around.

'I don't have it. My mum has it. She'll be here soon. She's just gone to get a coffee.'

'I can't give you your treatment without your Medicare card,' he grumbled.

'Do you have the methotrexate?' I asked, even though I already knew the answer.

'Of course I have the methe … metho …'

'Methotrexate,' I said, trying not to sound like a smarty-pants.

'You think you're clever then, do you?' he snarled.

I didn't know how to answer.

Mum, please hurry.

'Well, if you're so clever then, tell me your patient number. If you tell me your patient number, then I can give you your chemo.' He seemed delighted at the opportunity to trip me up.

I squeezed both of my teeny hands into fists and looked at a poster of a stunning white unicorn on the wall. I felt sorry for the unicorn. I'm sure it didn't want to be in here with the registrar who stank of onions and cabbage either.

'Two, zero, four, eight, three, six, eight,' I said.

'What?' he said gruffly.

'Two, zero, four, eight, three, six, eight,' I repeated. 'That's my number.'

'You know your number off by heart?' he asked sarcastically.

'Well, I've never thought about it before, but I think that's it. You can check it,' I suggested.

He turned his back to me again and flicked open my file. I kept my hands squeezed into tight balls.

'What do you think the number is?' he asked.

'Two, zero, four, eight, three, six, eight.'

'Well, clever Kirsty. Do I need to get a nurse to hold you down?'

'No.'

'I hope you don't kick me when I give you your injection. You're not going to cry, are you?'

'No.'

'All right then. Let's find a vein.' He did not wash his hands and he did not put on gloves. He put a tourniquet around my left wrist.

'Um … the veins are no good in my left hand. My right hand has the best veins,' I said.

He ignored me and pierced a cannula into the back of my left hand. He pulled it out and then pushed it back in, refusing to give up and creating stinging, screaming paths along my hand.

'You must have moved. I never miss,' he declared.

He pulled it out and then, using the same cannula, tried again. More zinging roads of pain wound their way inside my left hand. Never changing the cannula, he tried again and again and again.

'You must be moving. I'll try your right hand. This time, you need to stay still.'

He got it into the back of my right hand on the first attempt, taped the cannula in place and then turned to get the methotrexate. He stuck a syringe into the phial of hideously yellow chemo and sucked out the entire contents of the tiny bottle.

'I don't have the whole phial!' I exclaimed. 'I only have half of it and we throw away the other half!'

'Are you telling me that I don't know how to do my job?' He inserted the syringe into the cannula in the back of my right hand.

'NO! Please don't! Please just check the dosage!'

I'm about to be murdered with a methotrexate overdose.

The curtains around the treatment bed whooshed open.

'Mum!' There were tears in my throat, but not in my eyes. Mum was holding her cup of coffee.

'What's wrong, love?'

'He's going to give me the whole phial of methotrexate!'

Mum looked at the needle, poised and ready to be injected. 'Take it out! You'll kill her! She doesn't have the whole thing! Didn't you read her file?'

He unhooked the syringe and went over to check my notes.

Mum picked up my left hand. 'Oh my god, how many times did you try and get a needle into her?'

He didn't say a word, but squirted half of the contents of the syringe back into the small glass bottle and then came over and gave me the correct dose of chemo. He pulled the cannula out and gave me a cotton ball to press on the blood hole. His armpits smelled worse than the drugs. I thought nothing could smell more wretched than chemotherapy.

CHAPTER 13

One Last Flush

For over two years, my body was swamped with chemotherapy. My veins, barely clinging to existence, were injected over and over and over again. Down my gullet I swallowed thousands of pods of poisons. These tablets crawled down my oesophagus and into my belly, where my acidic tummy juices would make them erupt and dissolve and frolic into my bloodstream. My lower spine was invaded with the drugs designed to save my life. The shiny metal of needles, the yellow shades in a pile of pills and the maroon darkness of my blood all became so familiar. The sight of this arsenal had lost its ability to stun me. All these things had forced and forged a friendship with me. I needed a relationship with these objects in order to live and they needed a body to mould and merge with. I'd given poison a home.

No matter how sick I was I kept up with my schoolwork and went to school as often as I could. The thing I hated the most was having lumbar punctures in the land of screaming, Day Only.

Sometimes I would have treatment at 'clinic'. The space reserved for this was a room in the hospital that had no windows. It was a shadowy square with a large rectangular coffee table squatting in the middle of the room, surrounded by couches. The table was always covered in art and craft supplies — a well-intentioned attempt to distract us kids from our reality. There were all sorts of artwork on the brown walls: photographs of rainbows and waterfalls, and posters from cartoons and movies. Unfortunately, no poster and no amount of glitter and crayons could help any of us ignore a room full of bald heads and the smell of drugs that coiled up inside our nostrils.

A clinic day was what I considered an easy chemo day. Most of the time, the same two nurses — grinning, grandmotherly women — were the ones who gave you treatment at clinic. They were good at finding veins and if they ever missed getting one on the first go, a torrent of genuine apologies would fall upon you.

Mostly, I came to clinic for a 'flush of vincristine'. Vincristine always came in a fat syringe and looked like lemonade as it appeared to have bubbles in it, but they couldn't have been bubbles. When I say that syringe was fat, I mean it was *really* fat. It was thicker and longer than any banana you've ever seen.

Today was like any other clinic day. Another flush of drugs. Another flush of metal-mouth. Another step closer to being finished with all this nastiness. After today, I had one more flush left and the Prof said my treatment would be complete.

Once the nurse found a vein and inserted a cannula, she put on her spacesuit to protect herself and asked me for my full name and date of birth.

I answered.

'Do you have some jellybeans ready to go?' she asked.

'Yes,' Mum said, and she pulled a bag of jellybeans from her handbag and placed a white, green and pink jellybean (my favourites) in the palm of my free hand.

'Oh shit!' exclaimed the nurse from inside her astronaut attire. I giggled because I'd never heard her swear before. It sounded so dainty. 'Oh Kirsty, I'm sorry for cursing, but I've just realised I didn't put my glasses on.' She nodded towards a banged-up filing cabinet close by that was covered in faded stickers. Perched on top of the cabinet were her glasses. 'I'll have to take off all of this gear, get my glasses and then put on a new set of sterile gear. I'm sorry.' She went to remove the mask that covered her mouth.

'Wait!' I said. 'I can reach them and put them on for you.' I put my jellybeans on the treatment bed and reached for her glasses. I pulled her protective goggles up, put her glasses on and placed the goggles carefully back on top of her spectacles. 'Did I put them on all right?' I asked.

'Yes. That's perfect.' She picked up the monster-sized syringe and I popped the jellybeans into my mouth. 'Ready?' she asked.

I nodded.

She pushed the lemonade liquid into my vein. The chemo was cold from being in the fridge. A cold blast zoomed up my arm, and Mum began rubbing it with her warm hand. I chomped down on the lollies. The jellybeans did their best to shield my tongue from the full force of the vincristine, but it was too strong. An explosion of metal mixed with the taste of sugar flooded my mouth. Mum kept rubbing my arm, urging that horrid ice-spreading intensity to lose some of its power.

In the car on the way home, I could feel my blood begin to crackle and fizz like Fanta. The chemotherapy was spreading inside me. My blood became alert and adrenaline-charged because it knew the poison was powerful enough to kill it. Then it became thick and sticky like honey, too heavy to flow smoothly around my body. The chemo was part of me now. My body had to let it invade my cells, but not let it murder me. I've never felt anything else quite like it.

I tried to take slow deep breaths, but it's hard to breathe when your blood has become cement. Silently I wished for the chemo to work so I would never have to feel the snail-paced honey blood moving inside me ever again.

* * *

The last day of intravenous chemo had arrived. My spinal fluid and bone marrow were clear and I just had one more vincristine flush left to go on my treatment protocol. Mum drove through Brighton-Le-Sands so we could see the water on the way to Randwick.

'The water never looks the same.' Mum said this every time we drove this way to the hospital and she was right. Today the weather was overcast and the water looked navy-grey and choppy.

The Prof wanted to see me before my treatment so he could look at my blood on a slide under his microscope. Perhaps my blood knew today was the last day it had to be ravaged and was in a cooperative mood, because this time the pin-prick nurse had no trouble filling the tube. The Prof put a dark drop onto one of his glass rectangles. The glass clicked as he secured it in place under the microscope.

He stared at that drop for what felt like forever.

What can he see? What's he looking for? What if today isn't my last day of treatment?

Still looking into the microscope, he asked, 'What do we have you scheduled for today, Kirsty?'

He knew the answer and so did I, but I played along. 'Just a flush of vincristine,' I said, as my mouth and throat became a desert.

Something's wrong.

'You know what? I think we can skip the vincristine. I think you've had enough chemotherapy. I'm happy to finish your treatment today.'

Mum and I looked at each other to check that we'd both just heard the same thing. 'So, that's it?' asked Mum. 'She's finished treatment and we can go?'

'Yes,' he said, looking at us now and adjusting his half-moon glasses. 'Keep taking the tablets for the next few months and I'd like to see you in here in one month to check your blood, but yes, that's it. You can go home or go to school. You can go wherever you like.'

'Oh, that's great,' said Mum. She was so shocked her body wouldn't move. 'Thank you for everything.'

'My pleasure,' he said, smiling. 'Stay well and if you're worried about anything just give me a call.'

'Thank you,' I said.

I did it. I survived. I should do a cartwheel or something, but it's been so long I'm not sure my body can do them any more.

Mum had brought jellybeans for my vincristine flush, but now I could tell her to give them to Matthew as a treat after school. We didn't play any music on the way back to the Shire. We were both completely quiet until we came through Brighton-Le-Sands again.

'The water's changed,' said Mum. It was no longer a dreary, overcast day. The sun had squeezed through a crack in the clouds and sunlight stretched across the water all the way towards the horizon. The navy-grey water had transformed into a glimmering, glass-like turquoise.

'Where would you like to go?' she asked. 'We need to call your father, but after that, I'll take you anywhere you want.'

'Can I go to school?'

'Sure.'

* * *

Mum called Dad as soon as we got home. I couldn't hear what he was saying to Mum, but after a few moments she handed the phone to me. 'He wants to speak to you.'

'Hi Dad!' My voice was crackling with enthusiasm and joy.

'So … no more chemo,' he said.

'Yep.'

'I'm very proud of you. You'll have to give me an extra-special hug when I get home tonight and we'll have to have a fun day out to celebrate. I'll let you go so you can get to school.'

'Okay, bye Dad.'

It was about 11.30 by the time we got to school and there was an assembly going on, which meant there was hardly anyone around to tell our news to. We told the lady in the front office, who started crying and gave us both hugs. One of the Infants teachers was photocopying in the office and overhead the news.

'How do you feel?' she asked, seeming more excited than me and Mum.

'I don't know … good,' I said.

I don't know what I feel. I'm twelve years old and I've beaten cancer.

'I think we're in a bit of shock,' Mum explained. 'We were expecting to have one more round of chemo this morning, but they sent us home and told us she's finished treatment.'

I've finished treatment. I've finished treatment. I've finished treatment.

* * *

That weekend, Dad took our family and a whole bunch of our friends to Australia's Wonderland. Rollercoasters and dodgem cars seemed like a pretty good way to celebrate not dying. I'd start high school next year and I wouldn't be the girl at school with cancer any more. I'd just be a girl at school.

CHAPTER 14

The Pin-up Girl

I was in high school now. My hair was long enough for Mum to braid once again, and I was on a mission to live life to the max.

As soon as I started Year 7, I began to do everything. I signed up for classes in singing, debating, public speaking, dancing, acting and acrobatics — but not gymnastics. My Olympic opportunity had been stolen and destroyed by leukaemia, so the thought of doing gymnastics was just too painful. But it was okay because my weekends were now filled with theatre performances and events that helped young people with cancer.

I'll never forget the first event. Mum had spread word through the hospital newsletter that I did public speaking competitively and performed Shakespeare onstage and one weekend, the Prof asked me to come along to the University of New South Wales for an event supporting cancer sufferers and survivors. 'It's just a little get-together for patients and their families,' he said. I thought it would be good for Mum and Dad to go too. We never really talked about how we all felt when I was sick. It might be good for them to talk about it now that I was in the clear, with people who knew first-hand what they had gone through.

When we arrived, the Prof ushered me through a labyrinth of hallways and told me there were 'just a few people' who wanted to hear my story — about how I'd had cancer but was all better now. 'Would it be okay for you to just tell some people what you went through and what you're doing with your life now?'

'Sure,' I said.

He pushed open a set of double doors that opened into a huge lecture theatre. It must have had about two hundred seats in it, all of which were occupied. Scattered among the crowd were bald cancer kids.

The Prof stepped up to the lectern at the front and spoke. 'Thank you all for coming today. I'd like to introduce a special young lady that I know. Her name's Kirsty and I won't say anything else because I'll let her tell you about herself.'

Oh my goodness!

Thump thud. Thump thud. Thump thud. My heart muscle had never set a pace quite like this before. Some of the mums and dads were holding plastic vomit bags, ready and waiting for their child to spew at any moment. Even though we were at the university, the smell of cancer-town followed these families. My nose recoiled as I remembered when I smelled like that — a stew of antiseptic, tablets and possible death.

Thump thud. Thump thud. Thump thud.

I know exactly how every kid in this lecture theatre feels right now and I never want to feel it again. I want to live. I want to help. I need to speak.

And so I stepped in front of the lectern (it didn't feel right to stand behind it), my mouth opened and a steady stream of words trickled out.

'Good morning, everyone. I'll try to keep this short because looking around at some of you, I can see that you'd probably be a little more comfortable at home. I was diagnosed with cancer when I was nine years old and I'm now in remission and my life is the fullest it has ever been and I'm just as healthy now as I was before I got sick. I know when you're on chemo it's awful, but if I can get through it, then so can all of you.' I spoke for a little longer about how I kept up with my schoolwork while I was sick and about how good I felt now that I was better and then ... applause. Some parents were crying. My heart no longer thumped and thudded, it pitter-pattered.

I scurried over to Mum and Dad. Dad hugged me and whispered, 'I'm very proud of you.'

'But Dad, all I did was talk about myself ...'

'No, you did so much more than that.'

From that day onwards, I became the pin-up girl for cancer survival.

* * *

Who doesn't savour the crisp texture of a brand-new white t-shirt upon their flesh? I didn't even mind that it was big enough to fit a sasquatch. On the front of the shirt were the words 'I Support the Children's Leukaemia and Cancer Foundation'. Underneath these words was a cartoon of a young girl with pigtails doing cartwheels. On the back of the shirt, it read 'Why don't you?'

I couldn't think of a reason why not.

The early morning air made my nostrils sing. I adjusted the large t-shirt, tucking it into my black shorts in a useless attempt to make it look like it actually fit me.

I'd been asked by a man I'd never met to come and speak at an event called the Luke Savage Memorial Relay in Bundeena. Having made my debut at the university and been cast in the role of pin-up girl for cancer survival, I was now being asked to speak at fundraising events regularly. I never knew how people found me, but when this man rang the house, he said his name was Wayne and that the event was a running and walking race for the Children's Leukaemia and Cancer Foundation. He wanted me to speak and then officially start the race. Of course, I said 'yes'. I always said 'yes' if the aim of the event is to help anyone with cancer. I told him I wasn't a runner, but I'd like to compete in the walking section of the event. He seemed very happy about this.

On the appointed day, I looked for Wayne among a forest of lithe legs in fluorescent shorts. I needed to let him know I was here and ready to do whatever he needed.

'Kirsty?' a voice asked.

'Yep, are you Wayne?'

'Yes.' He shook my hand so hard I thought he might be planning on taking my arm with him. 'Thank you so much for coming along today.'

Wayne looked about the same age as my dad. He had blond hair and tanned skin. You could see how much time he had spent in the sun because tiny wrinkles splayed out of the sides of his eyes. Wayne, who I later learned was the founder and CEO of an event management business, had the same effect on people as a can of Red Bull. He kind of came over you like a sugary caffeine-injected rush and made you feel like you could achieve anything *and* do it with a grin on your face.

Gumtrees formed a tangled ceiling over us and cold dewy morning grass squished underneath everybody's sneakers. The long-legged strangers all grinned at me after I gave my pin-up girl speech. The local paper, the *St George and Sutherland Shire Leader*, snapped a photo of me beginning the race with a red-and-yellow horn. I walked the five-kilometre race, which took me through the bush, made me wade through a body of water that the runners simply strode through with their strong legs, then along the beach and back to where the race began. I came in first place of the walking division and ended up on the front cover of the *Leader*. The headline of the article was: 'At just 13, Kirsty truly is a lucky winner.'

More and more requests for events and articles came to me over the years and I did every single one of them, but my favourites were always the events with Wayne. He never told me what to say or how to say it. He never told me how long I should speak. He just told me to be myself and speak from the heart.

I remember someone once told me to stop smiling so much when I gave my speeches and asked me whether I could use my performance skills to pretend to cry, because it would make people feel sorry for me, and then they'd donate more money. I never did this. It would've been wrong and, besides, 'lucky winners' would never do such a thing.

CHAPTER 15

Remission Revelry

'Hey Kirsty, you perform in theatre stuff outside of school, right?' asked Ben.

'Yeah, why?' I said, as I dropped my school bag on the ground. I had met my friends Ben, Geoff and Debbie at our little spot, which was on a bunch of long metal bench seats on a large patch of lush grass overlooking our school's basketball courts and football field. There were humongous gumtrees overhead if you wanted shade, and if you wanted sunshine you just had to move down a few benches to soak up the hot rays. Today, we'd decided to sit on the sunny benches.

'When's the next performance?' asked Ben. His dark-brown hair was short and thick like steel wool, and made the green flecks in his hazel eyes more prominent. There was always a mischievous glint in his eyes.

'There's a show coming up in a few weeks. We're doing a play called *So Much to Tell You* by John Marsden and I'm playing this really nasty character called Kate. I even get to slap someone onstage. It's gonna be so much fun.'

I'd spent the last four years performing in amateur theatre productions. Mum and Dad had thought theatre would be good for me after being on chemo. They were worried I'd be too shy and would have trouble making friends when I started high school. Then they saw me in my first production — *A Midsummer Night's Dream*. Not only was I playing the coveted part of Puck, but, somehow, remnants of my gymnastic days remained and I was able to do a whole bunch of acrobatics on the stage.

The more time I was in remission, the longer my hair grew, and with every fundraising event where I was the face of cancer survival, the less worried my parents became. I was in Year 10 now and maybe it was the theatre, but there was no shortage of friendships in my life.

'We wanna come to the theatre,' said Geoff. I had christened him the BFG — Big Friendly Giant — as he towered over all of us at a whopping one hundred and ninety-four centimetres tall and, like Roald Dahl's character, he was a kind-hearted soul. He had spiky dirty-blond hair, which looked like the top of a pineapple from my perspective because I was so short.

'That would be awesome,' I said. 'Just make sure you sit up the back. I don't like seeing people I know in the front of the audience.'

'Sure, we can do that,' said Ben.

'Awesome,' I replied. I reached into my backpack and handed them both a flier with all the details of the performance. It was the end of the year. Next year we'd all be in Year 11 and school would begin to get serious, but for now, our crew was focused on having as much fun as possible and spending as much time together as we could.

We had our formal coming up and that was set to be a great night, especially since Ashley was going to host the afterparty, and everyone knew Ashley threw the best parties. His parents let him have friends over whenever he liked.

In primary school, I'd been the cancer girl, but in high school I was the academic girl, the theatre girl, the singing girl, the dancing girl, the acrobatic girl, the debating and public-speaking girl, the girl on the Student Representative Council, the girl who'd been skydiving and the girl who'd swum with sharks. I was the girl who did everything I could to make life full, because I'd learned something from being the kid with cancer — you've gotta pack your life to the brim with as much stuff that makes you happy as possible.

'Why the hell is everyone sitting in the sun?' With Jane's arrival, a grin couldn't help itself from bursting onto my cheeks. She sat down next to me, handing me two white bags of food from the canteen. Jane had luscious, long chocolate-coloured hair and skin like a porcelain doll.

'What's this?' I asked her.

'Food. Eat it,' she replied. She turned to Debbie, my best friend. 'So, Deb, have you asked Ashley to go to the formal with you yet?' Debbie had the best set of boobs I'd ever seen and dirty-blonde hair. She was stunning. We spent every spare minute together and many of those minutes were filled with discussions about how much she was in love with Ashley and his caramel-coloured shoulder-length hair.

'Yeah, Deb, have you asked him yet?' I chimed in.

'What if he says "no"?' Debbie, like any sixteen-year old, knew that rejection from someone you had a crush on was one of the most horrifying experiences one could endure.

'What if he says "yes"?' encouraged Jane. 'Listen, Deb, I'm going to ask Ben tomorrow. He gets to school early and so do I, so I'll ask him then. If he says "no", it's his loss. You need to do the same thing with Ashley.'

'I don't know,' said Debbie.

'You can do it, Deb,' I said. 'At least if you ask him, you'll know once and for all if he likes you.'

'Good point,' said Jane. 'If he says "no", then you can move on to somebody else and stop wasting your time thinking about him.'

'Okay,' said Debbie. 'I'll ask him, but only if Ben says "yes" to you. That will be a good sign that I should ask Ashley.'

Debbie was all about signs.

* * *

The Art Umbrella School of Performing Arts in Caringbah (affectionately known as the Art Brolly) was where I'd found a talented bunch of young people with whom I spent many hours rehearsing and performing. Four to six times a year, I'd take to the stage with individuals older and younger than me and from all walks of life. The theatre was safe for everyone. Not only did I have a collection of awesome friends at school, I also had a whole other bunch of friends from the Art Brolly.

Tonight, I had the privilege of performing in a play about a girl called Marina, who had horrifying burn scars on her face and is sent to a school where there are lots of nasty teenage girls who are mean to her because of her physical appearance. I was playing the part of Kate, who was the nastiest girl in the whole play. I had a scene where I said terrible things to Marina, and then I slap her. Ironically, the most beautiful girl at the Art Brolly was playing the part of Marina, but, with some clever prosthetics and make-up, half of her face was made to look like a mutilated mess.

It was our first performance and we'd never rehearsed the slap. As we all got ready backstage, this young actress said to me, 'When we have our scene, you can just hit me as hard as you like.'

'No way,' I said, 'you can't be serious.'

'Sure I am. Just hit me as hard as you want. It will look fake if we do it any other way.'

She was right. 'Okay, but I'll slap you on the arm. There's no way I'm slapping you across the face.' She did modelling part time and, even with the make-up and prosthetics giving her the illusion of being a burn victim, she was still breathtakingly gorgeous. Geoff and Ben would be so pleased they came along to support the arts tonight. In fact, there was always plenty of eye candy at the theatre school. Young models who needed to learn how to act would often join our class for a few months, and then I'd see them appear in television commercials and on shows like *Home and Away*.

I took rehearsals very seriously and always learned my lines off by heart long before most of the other cast. The curtain went up and I became Kate, the meanest girl in the school. I spat my venom at the other characters. I twisted my face in disgust at Marina's injured face and fearlessly stormed about the stage. It was great fun.

Then our big scene, nearing the climax of the play, arrived. 'You're an ugly, lazy, stupid pizza face!' I shrieked and swung my right hand, slapping Marina on the bare flesh of her upper arm. It made a terrific smacking sound and I heard the audience gasp with shock. I exited stage left and the scene ended. My hand was stinging from the slap.

'Oh my god, Kirsty! That really hurt,' the girl playing Marina quietly whispered backstage.

'I'm so sorry. I just got caught up in the scene. Are you okay?'

'I had no idea someone so small could be so strong.' She rubbed her arm where I'd hit her.

'I'm so, so sorry,' I pleaded.

'It's all right. It would've looked great for the audience.'

* * *

'Geez, Kirst! Did you really slap that chick onstage? It looked so real,' said Debbie after the show.

'Yeah, but she told me to do it,' I explained.

'That was actually pretty cool,' said Geoff.

'Yeah,' said Ben, 'I thought theatre was meant to be boring, but that was all right.'

'Thanks guys.' I beamed. 'Come on, I'll introduce you to some of the cast.'

CHAPTER 16

Boys and Slugs

Thumpety, thumpety, thump. My heart was ready to shatter my sternum. I took a deep breath in through my nose and, as I did, the nervousness surged through my core and charged my arms and legs with adrenaline. I needed something and my chances of getting it were rather slim.

My fate rested in the hands of one boy. In his company, my heart usually pounded loudly against my ribcage. But as hopeless as things seemed, I didn't have a choice. Only this guy could help me, so I walked towards him like I was getting ready to stand in front of the firing squad.

'What do you want?' snapped Brett from his spot on the lounge room floor. He didn't look up at me but remained fixated on the television screen. His strong hands shook the Nintendo controller as he rapidly pressed buttons, striving to win his game of *Mortal Kombat*.

'Um ...' I couldn't get my words out.

'You're not watching the TV. Mum said I'm allowed to play for as long as I want tonight.' His copper-coloured hair seemed to make him look even more hot-blooded than usual. It was as if his locks were flames of fire. The freckles on his face had vanished because he was so flushed from the effort of violently bashing imaginary characters.

I tried again. 'Well ...'

'Shit!' he yelled and the television screen displayed my fate in flashing lights.

GAME OVER!

'Brett!' called Mum from the kitchen. 'You can play for as long as you want, but *no swearing*!'

'Sorry, Mum!' Brett threw the controller down on the ground and stood up. He critically inspected my whole body, starting at my feet and making the journey up to my forlorn face. 'Why are you wearing a tight top? Are you trying to look sexy or something? Where are you going looking like that?'

'I'm going to Kathy's sixteenth birthday party. It's in Wollongong,' I said.

'Wollongong? How are you going to get there?' Suddenly, my tormentor realised exactly what I wanted from him. An evil smile crossed over his face. 'So ... you need a lift from your big brother.'

It was true. Dad and Matt had gone to the movies, Danielle was at her friend's place and Mum had said, 'I'm not sure about taking you all that way for a party. You know I see Kathy smoking cigarettes in Gymea all the time?' If Brett wouldn't take me, I wouldn't be going.

This was it — the moment of truth. 'Would you please drive me there and back?'

'Sure,' said Brett casually, and for a moment it was as if I'd been shot with a stun gun. 'There's just one thing you've got to do for me first.'

I put my hands on my hips. 'What do you want?' I was totally deflated and powerless, and Brett was relishing every second of my discomfort.

'All you have to do is say: "Brett is the best."' He grinned triumphantly.

'Brett is the best,' I mumbled.

'Sorry, I couldn't quite hear you. Do you think you could say it a little louder and clearer for me?'

'Brett is the best.'

About two hours later, Brett dropped me off at Kathy's party. He didn't utter a single word to me during the drive, but even if he had, I wouldn't have been able to hear him because he had Metallica playing as loud as the speakers would go the whole way there. As soon as I arrived, Kathy ran up to me, hugged me and took me straight into her laundry. Her laundry tub was filled with ice and booze.

Kathy had been my friend since the first day of kindergarten. I remember asking Mum how you made friends once you went to big school and she told me that it was easy, that all you needed to do was go up to someone, introduce yourself and ask them, 'Would you like to be friends with me?' I'd done exactly that on my first day of primary school, instantly becoming friends with Kathy and proving that Mum was right and that it was indeed very easy to make friends. Even though Kathy and I went to different high schools, we stayed in touch. We talked on the phone, wrote each other letters and were in the same singing classes after school. We'd even done a few performances together at Westfield shopping centre and in several competitions.

'All righty,' said Kathy, as she rummaged through the ice, 'what do you wanna drink?'

'Nothing,' I said.

Kathy stopped rummaging and looked annoyed. 'Everybody out there has a drink. You're already going to stand out because you're not from our school and you're the shortest person here. I really think you should have a drink.'

Her comment about my height sliced me like a paper cut across the back of my heels. Suddenly, I felt like I wanted to cry. I only really think about being short when people make comments about it. I had felt so genuinely happy lately that I hadn't thought too much about the fact that I would forever be vertically challenged because of chemotherapy. Although I was stuck at 144 centimetres for the rest of my life, I'd rather be short than dead. But remarks about my shortness were a disease I could not cure. What's strange is that I would never make a comment like, 'Geez, you're tall/fat/have a big nose,' but for some reason most people think it's fine to make comments about me being short.

Don't cry, I told myself. *Get a drink from Kathy and just hold it in your hand. You'll be fine. Smile. You've survived harder things than this.*

I sucked an extra dose of air into my nose. 'I'm not drinking beer. It's revolting.' The laundry tub was mostly filled with stubbies of VB.

Kathy pulled a green glass bottle out of the ice. 'Here. Strongbow. It's like apple cider.' She took off the lid and handed it to me. 'Take a sip,' she ordered.

I took a sip. 'Yuck!' My face contorted and crinkled as it went down my throat. It was like someone had mixed apple juice with nail polish remover.

She cracked open a stubbie of VB and handed it to me. 'Try this.'

'What?!'

'Trust me,' she said. 'Just take one sip.'

I did as she told me.

'Now take a sip of the Strongbow.'

I glared at her as I reluctantly sipped the Strongbow a second time.

'Now,' she said, 'which one tastes the most gross?'

'The beer!'

'Good! You'll take the Strongbow then.' She took the VB from me and guzzled it down herself. She pushed me out into the backyard.

Sitting at a picnic table was a group of teenage girls and guys. My eyes were pulled towards a boy with dark-brown hair. This guy had eyes that were so blue that they looked like small lights shining out of his face, and his skin was so tanned it was almost the colour of cocoa.

'This is Kirsty, my oldest and best friend in the whole world,' Kathy said, as she dumped her arm around my shoulders. 'She doesn't know anybody so make sure you're nice to her.' Then, from the depths of her backyard, the sounds of someone vomiting grabbed her attention. 'Daniel! What the hell?! I told you not to drink all of that Jim Beam!' Kathy hurried away.

The blue-eyed boy was looking at me now. I smiled and he smiled back.

'Hey everyone,' I said. 'You don't have to be nice to me just because Kathy told you to. You can get to know me first and then decide if I'm worth being nice to.'

The blue-eyed boy laughed. 'Sit down with us,' he said. He slid along the bench, making room for me.

Stay cool. Act normal. Don't say anything stupid, I instructed myself sternly. I sat down and took a sip of the sugary, acetone-tasting cider. The others were all drinking booze and some were smoking cigarettes. I made a mental note to take occasional sips of the Strongbow so it looked like I fit in.

After about an hour of small talk, the blue-eyed boy turned to me. 'Hey, I've noticed some things about you.' He spoke so quietly that I was the only one who heard him.

'Yeah?' I was trying to sound casual, but my voice sounded squeaky.

'The first thing I noticed is that you're really cute, and the second thing is that you've been holding on to the same drink for over an hour.'

Shit! The blue-eyed boy just told me I was cute. Wait! He's also noticed a flaw in my façade. I'm not drinking.

He continued looking me right in the eyes, which made me feel like I had popping candy fizzing and crackling inside my guts.

Argh! What do I do? Geez, this guy is really hot.

Honesty fell out of my mouth. 'I don't like alcohol, but Kathy made me drink this.' My hand reached for my locket and I squeezed it inside my fist.

I wonder if Melissa can see me now ... I know she'd tell me to not be so nervous just because a really hot boy is talking to me.

He grabbed the now-warm bottle of grog and proceeded to swallow the entire contents. He handed the empty bottle back to me. Nobody had seen what he'd done except me.

'You must really like Strongbow,' I said.

'Nope. It tastes like crap, but if Kathy comes over, she'll see you've drunk it.' He smiled at me again and his smile must have been magical because it forced a smile to spread across my cheeks too.

'Wanna go for a walk?' he asked.

'Sure.'

We went for a walk and I found out he liked to surf and ride his mountain bike, and that he played soccer and cricket. He asked me about what sport I did. I didn't tell him about my stolen dream to be an Olympic gymnast. I just told him I performed in theatre projects with the Art Brolly and that I was an acrobat. I told him I was also in the debating team at school, and did singing, dancing and public-speaking lessons. He clasped my hand and I flinched. I wasn't expecting him to touch me. No boys had touched me before. Well, unless you count Brett or Matt punching me in the arm when Mum wasn't looking.

He must have noticed, because he then asked, 'Is it okay if I hold your hand?'

I nodded way too enthusiastically.

Act normal. Just act like guys hold your hand all the time.

My stomach was swarming with flittering ladybugs and I reminded myself to breathe in and out. His hand felt big, smooth and warm and his palm wasn't sweaty, but I started to worry that soon my palm would be.

'Let's sit down,' he said, letting go of my hand and dropping down onto Kathy's front lawn.

I hesitated for a moment, standing over him.

'You can see more stars in Wollongong than you can in Kirrawee,' he said, as he turned his head up towards the sky.

I looked up. He was right, so I sat down next to him and we both gazed upwards together.

'I think I may be drunk,' he said. 'Is it just me or do those stars look like an apple?'

I started to giggle at him.

He put his arm around my shoulders.

The flittering continued in my stomach.

'Do you have a boyfriend?'

'No.' The ladybugs were blocking my throat. 'I'm too short.'

Why did you say that?

Before I could yell at myself any more, his face was pressed right up against mine. His lips were on my lips.

He's kissing me! What do I do?

My eyes were wide open, but his eyes were shut, so I shut my eyes too. His tongue was kind of pushing against my tongue. I opened my mouth wider. He seemed determined to explore the inside of my mouth.

This feels so slimy. His tongue feels like a determined warm slug poking in and around my mouth. I've dreamt about being kissed like in the movies for years, but this isn't right. This isn't like the movies.

My eyes fluttered open a few times, but his eyes stayed shut. He looked like he was sleeping and dreaming about something pleasant.

Do something! Copy what he's doing. This isn't a visit to the dentist, although my mouth is open so wide it kind of feels like it. How long does this last for? When do we stop?

I kept my eyes shut — I didn't want him to catch me with my eyes wide open — and I tried my best to copy what he was doing. Then, he just sort of stopped. He kissed me on the top of the head and hugged me with his long athletic arms. He smelled like Lynx body spray and saltwater. It felt nice to be hugged by a boy. I nestled my cheek against the soft woollen texture of his clean Quiksilver jumper. He was warm and I could hear his heartbeat. To my surprise, it was beating really fast.

Is he as nervous as me?

'You're a really good kisser,' he said softly into my hair. I cracked up laughing. He kept hugging me.

We kissed a few more times before Brett came to pick me up. I was slowly getting the hang of this kissing business, but it still felt weird to me. The movies made kissing look so soft and romantic, but it honestly felt like this boy liked me so much that he was trying to merge our bodies together using our mouths and tongues. It was as if he wanted to swallow my whole head.

I couldn't find Kathy when I left. Her comment about my height and her insistence that I drink alcohol had lacerated me, but the hugs and kisses from a very handsome guy made Kathy's remarks fade away into a dull ache.

I made sure my kissing instructor was far out of sight before Brett arrived to pick me up.

'So?' said Brett as I got into the car. 'How was the party? Your face looks weird.'

'The party was okay,' I replied, a thousand miles away. I kept thinking about all these random little details about the boy I'd just kissed — how he smelled like salty ocean water and Lynx body spray, how smooth his hands felt, how tiny my hand felt inside of his. I thought of the sound of his heart as it bashed against his ribs just from kissing me.

'"The party was okay,"' Brett mimicked and laughed. 'We're getting McDonald's on the way home.'

I didn't say anything back to him. I wanted to smile but tried not to in front of Brett. Then suddenly it dawned on me ...

What was the blue-eyed boy's name?! I just had my first proper grown-up kiss and I don't even know his name!

* * *

Ring, ring! Ring, ring!

'I'll get it!' I yelled at the top of my lungs and dashed for the phone in the hallway before anyone else could get to it. It wasn't a long dash, though, as I'd kind of been hanging around near the phone.

'Hello?' I did my best to not sound breathless, which is exactly what I was.

'Hi, it's Chris here. Could I please speak to Kirsty?'

Chris! His name is Chris! The blue-eyed boy has a name and it's Chris!

'Yep, I mean, hi. This is Kirsty.' I tried to sound as calm as I could, but it felt like my stomach was tripling in size and trying to leap out of my mouth.

'Hey, I hope you don't mind, I got your number off Kathy because I forgot to ask you for it last night.'

'That's okay.'

'I was just ringing to see if you wanted to go to the movies with me this afternoon.'

'Sure. That sounds good.'

Do I sound too excited? Does he know I've never had a guy ask me out before? Does he know he was my first proper grown-up kiss ever?

'I can meet you at Gymea and we'll head to Miranda. Do you want to see *Men in Black*?'

He sounds so calm. He doesn't sound nervous at all. He's definitely way more experienced with this stuff than I am. What if he wants to have sex? I don't think I'm ready to have sex. I'm not really interested in Men in Black. *Isn't that some alien movie with Will Smith? That's not really my kind of movie.*

Who cares? I'll be too nervous to pay attention to the movie anyway.

'Yeah, I can meet you at Gymea,' I said, trying to sound bored with the conversation. 'What time?'

'Is two o'clock okay with you?'

How come he sounds so relaxed? This guy must be a player. I must be just one of the many girls he's hooked up with.

'Two o'clock is fine,' I said.

'Cool. I'll see you then.'

Is that a smile I can hear in his voice?

'Great ...' *Don't linger. Get off the phone before he discovers how nervous you are.* 'Bye.'

'See you soon,' he said and I quickly hung up.

CHAPTER 17

Cancer Stamp

'Mum? I met a guy at Kathy's party and he asked me to go to the movies with him. Is that okay?'

'Oh!' said Mum. She seemed shocked. 'I'm not so sure, love … How well do you know him? You only just met.'

I had anticipated Mum's reluctance and caution. This guy was a stranger to her, and to me really, but I just wanted Mum to let me go without questioning me.

'Well, he goes to school with Kathy.' This fact wasn't going to help my cause. Mum had never been a huge fan of Kathy. I quickly went on. 'He's in the same year as me at school. He's into surfing just like Dad and he plays lots of sport. It will still be daytime when we go to the movies …'

'Oh, all right then. Make sure you're home by six o'clock. So, is he your boyfriend?' Mum asked.

'I don't know, Mum. He didn't ask me to be his girlfriend or anything, he just asked me to go to the movies with him.'

'Oh, okay. I don't know how people your age do things. Maybe he thinks you're his girlfriend?'

Am I his girlfriend? How will I know? I definitely can't ask.

'Just make sure you know where you stand,' advised Mum.

I nodded in exaggerated agreement with her. Before she could say any more, I slipped back into my bedroom to count down the minutes until I left for my first proper date with a boy.

* * *

I arrived early at Gymea station, but I'm always early. I sat on a bench and waited.

What if he doesn't show up?

It felt like my head was no longer attached to my neck and had popped off into the air.

Breathe. Control yourself. You've handled cancer. You can handle a date at the movies.

'Hey.' He'd arrived.

'Hi!' I said. *Stay cool*, I ordered myself.

We started to walk along the Kingsway towards Miranda. We were both silent.

Say something! Please say something.

'So,' he said. Just to hear him say that one word made delight ooze down to my toes. 'I heard something about you.'

'Oh yeah?' I said, trying to sound unfazed. 'Who did you hear it from?'

'Well, when I rang Kathy to get your phone number, she told me you had cancer when you were in primary school. Is it true?'

My stomach dive-bombed into my knees. My heart felt like it was a cinder block. One tear plopped down onto my cheek, but Chris didn't see it. My face filled with flames of fury. *Kathy, why would you tell Chris? My first date ever and I feel like I'm the freak back in the school playground.*

'Yeah, it's true,' I said. 'Is that a problem?' It felt like my anger was seeping through to my words, but I tried not to sound angry because I wasn't angry at him. I prepared to turn around and walk home by myself.

'No!' said Chris. 'It's not a problem. Kathy just said that's the reason why you're so short … because you had cancer and it made you stop growing normally.'

'Is the fact that I'm short a problem?' My words were laced with venom, but to this day I still don't know if Chris picked up on the pain in my words.

'No,' said Chris. 'I just wasn't sure if Kathy was telling the truth. I think you're really sexy.'

His hand reached down and grabbed my hand. It felt just as enchanting as it did the first time he held my small fingers inside his big, tanned hand.

'Sorry, I didn't mean to sound like an arsehole,' he continued. 'You look really healthy to me, so I didn't know whether to believe Kathy or not.'

My stone heart dissolved into liquid as the cosiness of his hand gripped mine.

'I'm really sorry,' he said.

I abruptly realised we had stopped walking and were facing each other. It felt like a stand-off. Part of me wanted to let go of his hand, walk away and never look back, but another part of me told me to take a deep breath and go to the movies with Chris, the hot, shiny-eyed boy who told me I was sexy. It's what Melissa would've wanted me to do.

'It's okay,' I said. 'We better start walking if we want to make it to the movie on time.'

We set off again, holding hands, and he began to tell me about how he'd gone surfing that morning and how he wanted to go to the beach with me soon. We saw *Men in Black* — well, that's what was playing on the screen, but we were too busy kissing to follow the storyline.

Kathy had stamped me as 'the short cancer girl', but Chris had stamped me as 'the cute and sexy girl', so did Kathy's stamp really matter?

CHAPTER 18

Splash-a-thon

I inhaled the fresh morning oxygen. Towering gumtrees occupied the car park with their vast trunks, their ancient arms looming protectively over me and my family. As our feet crunched along the gravel in the car park, I could hear my thongs smacking against my heels. We walked under the metallic-blue banner that was displayed over the automatic doors of the Sutherland Leisure Centre. We went down a few stairs and another automatic door swung open instantly, urging us to come in. The intense smell of chlorine and bleach was so overwhelming it made me giddy for a few moments. We approached the counter in the foyer of the leisure centre and I dropped my backpack at my feet. Shades of blue were everywhere. The foyer was painted blue, the carpet was aqua blue, the railings and all the fixtures were sky blue, and the turnstiles that pushed you inside the centre were navy blue.

This was a preview for the teal-coloured fifty-metre lap pool inside the centre.

'Can I help you?' asked the woman behind the counter, who was wearing a blue polo shirt.

'We're here for the Splash-a-thon today for the Children's Cancer Institute of Australia,' I said.

'Oh, wonderful,' the woman replied. 'Just go straight on through to the outdoor pool.'

I heaved my backpack onto my shoulder. A few more steps, and we were standing outside on squishy bright-green grass. The grass at the leisure centre was never dry and it never had bees or bindies. Palm trees were dotted around the pool that my friends and family and I would spend the next nine hours swimming laps in to raise money for cancer research.

This was an event organised by Wayne, so I already knew it was going to be an awesome day. It was the third year in a row that this event was running, and it grew bigger every year. The way the Splash-a-thon worked was that you needed a team of at least ten people who would take it in turns swimming laps in the pool for nine hours. Even though it wasn't a competition, the event always drew lots of athletes, who'd try to swim the most laps or practise for upcoming triathlons or even just try to beat their personal-best times. But the point of the event, and indeed most of the events that I did with Wayne, was for people to be active, raise some money and have fun. My dream was to one year be the team that raised the most money.

We walked down the grassy hill and onto the orange-brown concrete path. In bright-yellow paint, every few metres, the following words were painted in big capital letters: DO NOT RUN. We followed the path to the giant cement steps at the shallow end of the pool, with its shimmering inviting water and its white, red and blue lane ropes. I put my things down in front of the lane that was meant for our team. This was where we'd all be hanging out for the day.

'G'day, Kirsty,' a familiar, joy-filled voice said.

'Hey, Wayne,' I said.

'Where's my hug?'

I promptly threw my arms around his middle. Wayne wrapped his toned arms around my head and shoulders, squeezing me too hard into his chest, and then he put his chin on the top of my head. He was a similar hugger to my Dad — he hugged you like he meant it.

'How are ya?' he asked, releasing me from his tight grip.

'I'm good. How are you?'

'I'm fantastic. Today is going to be such an amazing day. All week those clouds have been bugging me, but we got here this morning and suddenly, geez, I wish you'd been here to see it, it was like the clouds parted right over the pool. Hi, Jill,' he said, as he gave Mum a peck on the cheek. 'Good to see you here, Peter,' he said, as he shook hands with Dad.

Brett was sulking about giving up his day for charity, so he ignored Wayne, focusing all his attention on his Gameboy, but

Matt, mimicking the men, grabbed hold of Wayne's hand and shook it firmly. Wayne, Mum, Dad and I laughed. Danielle was in America working at a camp for adults with disabilities. She was due home before Christmas.

'Heaps of my friends are coming today and we've raised about two thousand dollars,' I proudly informed Wayne.

'That's fantastic. Listen, I've gotta go and do a couple of things, but we've got nine hours here today, so I'll catch you around, all right?'

'Yeah, of course, go and do what you need to do,' I said.

'I'm so glad you can all be a part of this.' He pulled me in for another hug and smacked a big wet kiss on my forehead. 'Look at that,' he said, pointing up at the sky, 'nothing but sunshine. We couldn't have wished for a better day than this.'

I sat down on the jumbo-sized cement steps to wait for the rest of my team: Geoff, Jane, Ben, Debbie, Ashley and Jake. Jake was new to our group at school. He had long blond hair and braces. When Debbie had told him about the event today, he was very keen to join our swimming team. I put on my sunglasses, flopped my hair to one side, closed my eyes and revelled in the searing sun as it baked new freckles onto my face.

Gosh, it's good to have hair and to be sitting in the sun surrounded by family and friends. The summer holidays are coming up and I can't wait until the end-of-year formal next weekend.

Over the next few minutes, all my friends arrived. The pool was crowded with about one hundred people who were all here for the event.

'Attention, everyone.' Wayne's voice boomed over the loudspeakers. 'If I could just have everyone's attention … Thank you all for coming to this event. Some of you would have come to this event when it was a fundraiser for the Children's Leukaemia and Cancer Foundation. The foundation has a new name; it's now the Children's Cancer Institute of Australia, but its aims are the same — to minimise the suffering for children with cancer and one day find a cure, so no child has to endure this horrific illness.

'Now, in lane three we have a very special girl with a very special team.'

I froze. I knew what was coming and it always made me squirm.

'That very special girl is Kirsty. Now, not all of you know Kirsty. Kirsty, can you just give us a wave?'

With a crooked smile planted on my face, I waved. Every person at the event was looking right at me. My friends all grinned.

'I think it's important for us to remember that we are here today helping real people, just like Kirsty, by raising money for the Children's Cancer Institute of Australia. Kirsty, can I get you to come up here real quick and say a few words?'

Here I was again, in the role of survivor, trying to make all the pain mean something beyond myself. I walked up to Wayne and his loud microphone. I inhaled and nerves charged my arms and legs.

Kirsty … this is not about you. This is for charity. Don't be such a baby.

I clutched my silver locket and the words tumbled towards the crowd.

'I just want to take this opportunity to thank everyone for being a part of this event today. I was diagnosed with cancer when I was nine years old and had two and a half years of chemotherapy. If it wasn't for the work and research of the Children's Cancer Institute of Australia, I may not be alive. I'm sixteen years old and I've been in remission for over four years now …'

Suddenly, loud applause began to sound from all around me. I guess people thought being in remission for over four years was worth clapping about. My friends joined in, whooping and whistling and making as much noise as they possibly could.

Geez, all I did was have cancer as a kid. This is so bizarre. I'm just me. I'm not sure I should be clapped about. It's not like I chose cancer. It chose me.

I felt so awkward, but I smiled. The applause and cheering died down. I continued.

'I'm really lucky that I was able to survive, but my friend Melissa and lots of other kids die from cancer and …' I faltered.

'… it's important that we keep raising money for the Children's Cancer Institute of Australia so that no kid has to die from cancer.'

Applause broke out again.

'Thank you for sharing that with us, Kirsty,' said Wayne. 'Isn't she special?'

Oh geez, Wayne …

I had completed my duty as spokesperson for cancer survival and all I had to do now was enjoy the day.

* * *

'Look at this!' Jane exclaimed. She had been handed a bright-green bathing cap and was looking quite repulsed.

'Sorry guys, it's the rules of the event,' I said. 'When you're in the water swimming laps, you have to wear our team's bathing cap.'

'We'll all look like we're wearing condoms on our heads,' Jane grumbled.

I pulled my favourite white t-shirt off my head and, as I did so, a gigantic wave of insecurity washed over me. Like most sixteen-year-old girls, I didn't exactly love my body. I sucked in my white tummy as I proceeded to tie double knots in my aqua-blue bikini top.

Suddenly I realised that Jake was looking at me. As I tied my long hair into a bun and yanked that green bathing cap onto my head, Jake's eyes were scanning my whole body. I could feel where his eyes moved from my feet, up my legs and onto my tummy. It felt so strange.

Why is he looking at me like that?

'You should take off your board shorts and just wear your bikini in the water,' advised Debbie.

'I don't know …' I said.

'The bikini suits you, Kirst. Just pull down your pants,' Jane urged. 'If I had your little body instead of my fat arse, I'd probably walk around naked.'

My heart went *rat-a-tat-tat* as I started to pull down my board shorts. I tried to look like I didn't care, but I cared. I really, really cared.

'Good girl. Get your clothes off.' Jane laughed at her own joke.

I wish no one would ever look at me.

I slid into the pool. The coolness of the water gave me a burst of fresh energy. I swam up and down the fifty-meter pool for close to an hour, and then it was Jane's turn.

'Get out of my way!' boomed Jane at a couple of small children as she got into the pool. The children scurried out of that pool faster than a couple of rats off a sinking ship.

'Hey, Jane,' I said, 'those kids are sharing our lane with us today. They're from Laguna Street Public School in Caringbah and they usually raise more money than any other team that swims in this event. Their whole school helps raise money.'

'Well, they need to learn to respect their elders and get out of my way when I tell them to!'

We all laughed as Jane pulled her goggles down onto her face. She looked like a furious googly-eyed frog with her green bathing cap and bad attitude.

'Do they get anything for raising the most money?' asked Jake.

'Nah,' I said, 'but I guess they get the satisfaction of knowing they beat all the adults.'

'Well, it would be easier to raise money if you had a whole school helping you out,' pointed out Debbie. 'And people don't say "no" to little kids who ask for money for charity. Those kids have an unfair advantage.'

'We should get our school to help raise money next year,' said Ben.

'Yeah,' I said, impressed, 'we should do that.'

'We can't let a bunch of little kids beat us,' said Jane. Then she pushed herself off.

'Hey Kirst,' said Debbie, 'wanna come for a walk with me to the bathroom?'

'Sure,' I said.

We walked to the toilet block, but just before we went inside, Debbie grabbed my arm and pulled me behind a vending machine.

'What's going on?' I said. 'I thought you wanted to go to the bathroom.'

'Nope. Geoff told me something and I had to tell you.'

'Okay ... what is it?'

'Jake has a crush on you!' She delivered the news in a high-pitched squeal.

'Yeah, right.' I went to walk off, but Debbie pulled me back.

'I'm being serious. He told Geoff that he thinks you're beautiful and you should've seen his face when you were giving your speech to the crowd. He's totally into you, but he's already asked this girl, Sarah, to go to the formal with him and he knows you have something going on with Chris, because they play soccer together.'

I was stunned. Several girls in our year at school had crushes on Jake. He looked like your very stereotypical long-haired surfer kind of guy, but he was also an amazing artist who was always sketching these highly detailed drawings in class. He was very popular.

'I don't know what to say,' I said, shaking my head in disbelief.

'This is awesome! You've got two guys who are fully into you. Geoff wanted me to find out if you liked Jake, but I told him you're with Chris.'

'Good. I *am* with Chris. He's so handsome and I love going to the beach with him. He's a really good guy.'

'This is so exciting! This usually only happens in the movies! It's like a love triangle!' Debbie jumped up and down and I laughed at her.

'I think that's taking it bit far.'

'Well, Geoff wanted me to tell you and I have, so my work here is done.' She beamed at me.

'All right. Let's get back to everyone.'

I can't believe it. Two guys liking me at once. Melissa would love to be in my shoes, but I don't know about this. If Jake knows I'm seeing Chris and he's bringing a date to the formal, why would he even say anything to Geoff? This seems a bit wrong.

* * *

Laguna Street Public School raised the most money at the Children's Cancer Institute of Australia's nine-hour Splash-a-thon in November 1997. But my friends were now hungry to be the team that raised the most in 1998.

'So, Kirst, we'll definitely get together for this thing next year?' asked Ben.

'Sure. As long as you guys are keen to do it again?'

'Hell yeah!' exclaimed Jane. 'Then we can teach those Laguna Street kids what it feels like to lose.'

CHAPTER 19

Buggers

My hair was a sculpture of immaculate curls, held together by bobby pins and hairspray. I was wearing my first-ever pair of heels — black satin wedges. Of course, my only accessory, snug inside her silver, heart-shaped home around my neck, was Melissa. A friend of Mum's had carefully measured my body and sewn me a red gown especially for the occasion. The night of the Year 10 formal was here.

We squished into the limo that we'd all chipped in for. Jake and his girlfriend, Sarah, sat next to me, and Ben, Jane and Geoff sat in front of me. Jake's back was pushing against me as he sucked on Sarah's face all the way from Kirrawee to Cronulla. The only noise in the back of that limo were their sloppy kisses. I stared uncomfortably into my lap, only glancing up at Ben and Geoff for a few seconds to see if they were squirming as much as I was. As soon as my eyes met Ben's, he pulled a silly face at me, raising his eyebrows. Geoff poked his tongue out and mimed kissing an invisible girl next to him. I stifled a giggle, fiddled with my locket and looked back down at my lap.

* * *

We had arrived at the function hall in Cronulla. There were long tables covered with white tablecloths and yellow roses had been placed in vases in the middle of each table. All the tables surrounded a diamond-shaped dance floor.

'Get a photo of me and Ashley,' Debbie instructed me. Debbie, with a nudge from Jane and myself, had asked Ashley to be her date and he had said "yes". Ben was Jane's date. She'd asked him just like she said she would, so Debbie had had to follow through and ask Ashley. There wasn't enough room in our limo so I'd decided not to bring Chris along as my date.

As the flash went off on my camera, I felt a pain like an invisible crone had scraped her fingernails across my spine. The pain was so sharp that it forced me to collapse into a chair. Not wanting to alarm anyone, I remained seated and sipped on some water. The song 'My Sharona' began pumping. Everybody was getting up to dance.

'Kirst! It's your song!' Debbie yelled.

'Are you gonna come and dance?' asked Jane.

Shit … I'm not sure if I can stand up.

Debbie grabbed my arm and pulled me to my feet. The pain in my lower back intensified, but somehow I managed to walk towards the dance floor with my friends.

Oh, please let this go away … This can't be …

To my alarm, right in front of Sarah, Jake grabbed hold of my hands and started to dance with me. In a matter of seconds, I pulled away from him. 'It's too hot to dance!' I yelled over the music. I began weaving my way through the writhing bodies of my friends back to our table.

* * *

Debbie and I had told our parents we were sleeping over at Jane's house after the formal. It wasn't a complete lie. We would be sleeping at Jane's … eventually. We were just making a slight detour to Ashley's house for the afterparty. We all gathered in the backyard. Ashley had set up a giant circle of folding camp chairs. It was like alfresco dining, but there was no food, just an old wooden table with bottles of booze and a big blue esky with cans of soft drink in the middle of the circle. This was the usual set-up at Ashley's parties. He also had a huge grassy backyard so there was plenty of room for everyone.

'Do you want a Bombora and lemonade?' asked Jane.

'I don't really like alcohol,' I said, remembering how Kathy had forced me to drink. I hadn't really spoken to Kathy since her party. The things she told Chris about me still stung. I saw

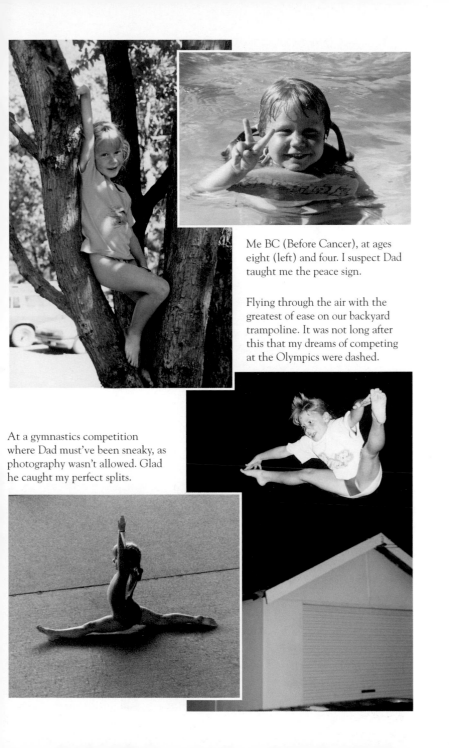

Me BC (Before Cancer), at ages eight (left) and four. I suspect Dad taught me the peace sign.

Flying through the air with the greatest of ease on our backyard trampoline. It was not long after this that my dreams of competing at the Olympics were dashed.

At a gymnastics competition where Dad must've been sneaky, as photography wasn't allowed. Glad he caught my perfect splits.

The day the Prof got me to school on time for school photos. The Band-Aid on my right arm is from the blood test he gave me.

One of my first celebrity meetings while on treatment was with Noeline Donaher, from the TV show *Sylvania Waters*. She was absolutely lovely. Note my hair trying to grow in between rounds of treatment.

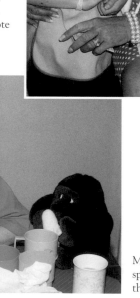

Me wearing the sparkly rainbow hat that Mum got for me.

A chemo day in clinic with the bubbly grandma-like nurses. The woman on the right is wearing one of the free wigs donated to the hospital that I did *not* want.

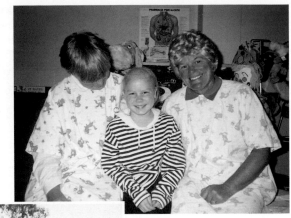

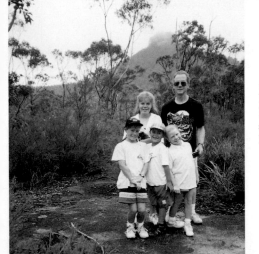

(Clockwise from top left) Danielle, Dad, me, Matt and Brett on our camping trip. We're about to climb Pigeon House Mountain.

A fully healthy, in-remission me in Year 9 with long hair all grown back and shining in the sun. Here I am with my siblings, Matt (left), Danielle and Brett.

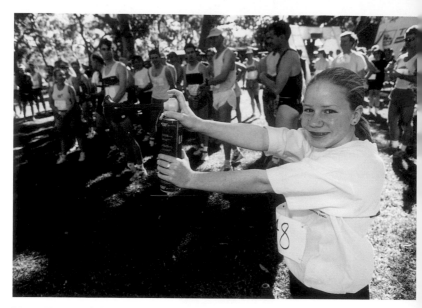

Me, in Year 8 with braces, being the pin-up cancer girl at the Luke Savage Memorial Relay in Bundeena. (*The St George and Sutherland Shire Leader*)

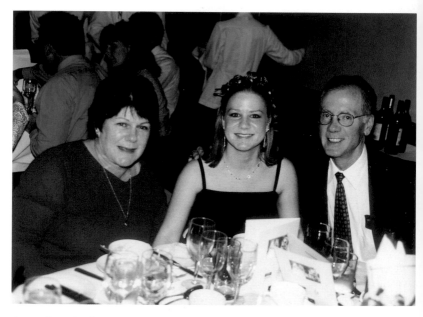

A very fancy fundraising event for the Children's Cancer Institute of Australia, where I gave a speech. Mum and Dad were right there with me. I was in remission.

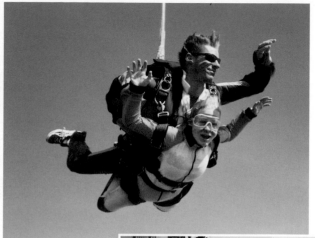

I lived life to the fullest in the four years when I had a reprieve from cancer. Here I am at sixteen years old, only a few months away from relapse, and skydiving in Cairns.

During remission and after relapse, theatre became a big part of my life. Here's the Art Brolly (Art Umbrella School of Performing Arts) crew. I'm the one in the middle with the grey hoodie, back on chemo and with strange fuzzy hair trying to grow between treatments.

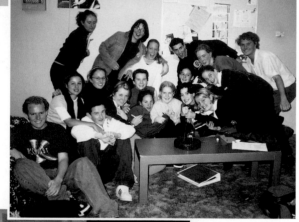

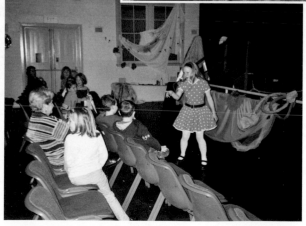

Theatre remained a love of mine long after high school. Back to being a healthy me at age twenty-one, here I'm at a dress rehearsal for *Alice in Wonderland*.

Big bunch of fairies splash out in swim marathon

By BRAD FORREST

ONE girl checked herself out of hospital to swim.

Another swam for the whole nine hours.

And ordinary people joined the celebrities and stars to earn more than $40,000 for the Children's Cancer Institute of Australia at the annual Nine Hour Marathon Splash at Sutherland Leisure Centre on Saturday.

More than 40 teams of swimmers took part in the all day swim and fun day.

Marathon swimmers like David O'Brien, Des Renford, Baden Green, Steve Yates and Peter Tibbitts were there.

They were joined by other teams, including stars like Commonwealth

Games gold medalist Simon Cowley, who was "crash tackled" by St George league captain Mark Coyne.

Cronulla league stars Dean Treister and Brett Howland joined in the fun, along with Sydney Kings' big man Dean Utoff as little children were entertained away from the water by centre staff in and around the sand pit.

A former policeman from the district came down with a team from Queensland's Sunshine Coast to help out.

But it was two young ladies who stood out in their fundraising efforts.

Catherine Allen decided to swim for the

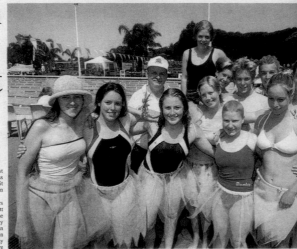

■ THE biggest fundraising swim team, the Water Fairies. led by leukemia patient Kirsty Everett (middle front), during the nine-hour splash.
Photo: LISA McMAHON

whole nine hours, from 9am Saturday until 6pm.

And after checking herself out of hospital, gutsy leukemia patient Kirty Everett – a regular at these days – led the Water Fairies team in

raising more than $4000 through their swimming effort.

It was the most raised by any team on the day.

At the end of it all, a happy and hard-working organiser, Wayne Staun-

ton, proudly announced more than 1000km had ben swum by 45 teams.

"And that's given us more than $40,000 to bank for the cancer institute," he added.

The Water Faeries after raising the most money at the splash-a-thon, as I promised we would. I made sure to cover up my portacath with my blue Mambo bathing suit.
(*The St George and Sutherland Shire Leader*)

Will see Sue in morning about pain maybe all this is due to Dexamethadine steriod. Kirsty didn't have L-asparaginase today.

Day 24 Thurs 19-2-98. (Hospital Stay)

Kirsty woke up few times in night to go to toilet, still pain in chest, Kirsty is still very low hurts to move, pain in chest and all over, Alex & Joseph saw her will have x-ray on chest to see what is causing pain again! Alex came to see her, will give some morphin for pain.

To Kirsty much love!

[Olivia Newton-John signature]

Day 25 Frid 20-2-98 (Hospital) Alex, Joseph and Sue saw Kirsty today maybe will check bone-marrow if counts are good will have chemo today, pain in back & chest is better but still there. Sue will see us before lunch. Lydia rang & Kaye from Suth Hosp school came in to see us. It is 10-50am Kirsty is feeling itchy from morphin. Had bone-marrow & lumbar punct at 3-15- 3-30pm Kirsty went well. Sue, Alex & Joseph came said the marrow wasn't a good take but wants to press ahead with chemo on Saturday. Sue seems quite concerned about Kirsty tolerance of chemo.

Mum kept a diary and wrote an entry every day that I was on treatment. This page was autographed by Olivia Newton-John the day she came to visit the hospital.

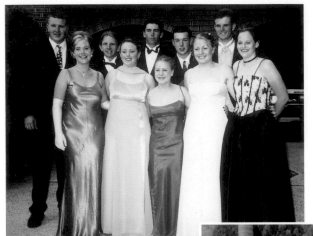

The Year 12 formal, which I attended as well as helped organise. Jane is in the black-and-white dress, Geoff is at the far left, Ashley is next to him, and Ben is just over my left shoulder.

Me and Debbie, the quintessential best friend, the night of the Year 12 formal. I wore fairy wings, as fairies had become an intense obsession for me after one manifested itself in the tub.

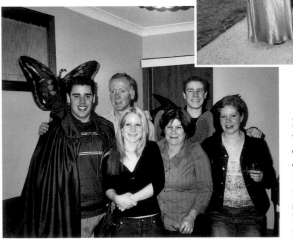

My twenty-first birthday, where the theme was to come as a non-human creature of some kind. Here I am, a healthy me, two-time cancer survivor, and I couldn't have done it without my family. We did it.

her at singing classes, but didn't stick around and speak to her like I always used to.

'Here, have a sip of this and if you like it, I'll pour you one. If not, I'll give you a cup of lemonade.'

I accepted the small white plastic cup. It smelled like lemons and coconut. 'Wow,' I said, surprised by the deliciousness of the scent. I took a small sip. It didn't even taste like alcohol. 'Oh my gosh, Jane! It's nice. I've never tasted alcohol that I actually liked before.'

'I'll pour you one,' she said.

'Don't put too much Bombora in it.'

Jane dropped a tiny dash of the coconut-scented liquid into a plastic cup for me. 'It's not even enough to get Thumbelina drunk,' she said. We both laughed. 'Cheers, big ears!' We tapped our cups together and sipped our drinks.

Geoff and Ben came over to sit with us.

'Who wants to learn how to waltz?' Ben asked.

'Teach Kirsty,' said Jane, pushing me towards him. Even though he was Jane's date, since asking him to the formal Jane had decided she had a crush on a guy in Year 12 at school. She had told Debbie and me that Ben was 'too much of a boy for her' and that she 'wanted a man'. But her crush had no idea she even existed (yet), so she had kept her plans with Ben.

'Stand on my feet,' he said.

'My dad used to get me to do this when I was a little girl,' I said.

'I'm not your daddy,' said Ben.

I held on to Ben and he held on to me as I positioned my feet on top of his feet and he started dancing around.

Jake approached us. 'What's going on here?'

'Ben's teaching me how to waltz. Where's Sarah?' I asked.

'She went home. I just broke up with her,' said Jake.

'Seriously? The two of you were all over each other in the limo,' remarked Jane.

'Yeah, I know. Something didn't feel right and I think I like someone else.'

'Who?' asked Jane.

'I'll let you know once I'm sure,' said Jake, as he stared intently at me with a look I couldn't decipher.

Ben and I continued dancing. Then Debbie came running up to us, grabbed my arm and steered me away from everyone.

'Ashley kissed me!' she squealed.

'Let's jump up and down,' I said and we held tightly onto each other's forearms and began jumping up and down on the spot. Whenever something exciting happened, Debbie and I would take a moment to embrace the joy of the situation with this mini ritual. When I told her about Chris kissing me for the first time, her response was, 'We need to jump up and down over this.'

'Tell me the details,' I urged her.

'Well, I just went up to him to say "hello" and so he knew I was here and he just grabbed me and said, "You look really beautiful tonight," and then he kissed me, like, right on the lips!'

'Oh my gosh! Did he put his tongue in your mouth?' I asked.

'No, it was just a kiss right on my lips. No tongue, but he kind of lingered as he did it. Eeeee!' Deb shrieked with joy. 'This is a sign! He'll definitely ask me to be his girlfriend.' Deb began jumping up and down again, so of course I joined in. 'This is the best night of my entire life.'

I wanted it to be mine too. But my attention was torn between my friends and the growing dull throb in my lower back, which was starting to return.

At first, it was just a low pulse, and then the throbbing grew stronger and it took a great amount of effort to stand up. I went and found a lush patch of grass in Ashley's backyard. I just needed a few minutes and a few deep breaths on my own. I plonked down, cross-legged, on my bottom. The grass came up to my knees, so it was well overdue for a good weekend mowing.

Oh my god … I can feel something so wrong twisting my insides.

'Are you all right, Kirst?' asked Geoff, towering over me before sitting down on the ground beside me. Then Jake came over, and Debbie, and Ben and Jane. I swallowed my frustration that they had followed me out here, even though I was trying to get away from them.

I can't tell them what's going on, can I?

'I don't know,' I said. 'I don't feel so good. I've got this really bad pain in my back.'

'It might be from wearing high heels all night,' offered Debbie optimistically.

'No … I think it's something worse. I think …'

It's coming back. The cancer pain.

'Do you ever worry about getting cancer again?' asked Jake.

'Not usually, but — I don't know … this pain in my back … it's so strong. I haven't had anything like this since I was a kid on chemo. Cancer survivors get phantom pain sometimes. Our bodies remember the agony they once felt. I'm hoping that's it.'

'Do you have to go for check-ups at the hospital?' asked Ben.

'Yeah, I'm meant to go on Monday. I only go once a year. They'll do a blood test and check everything's okay.'

'I'm sure you'll be fine,' said Jane. 'You'll feel better once you've had the test and get the results and I bet everything will be okay.'

'Yeah … I hope so.'

'We'd better start walking back to my place,' said Jane. 'I bet Ashley's mum wants to get some sleep.'

'I don't wanna go,' said Debbie. 'It's been such a good night that I don't want it to be over.'

'Why don't you sneak back here at 4 am and we'll meet up out on the street so we don't wake Ashley's mum?' Ben suggested. Ben, Jake and Geoff were sleeping over at Ashley's place.

'Really?' Debbie clearly liked Ben's plan. 'Will you make sure Ashley comes out?'

'Sure.' The pact was made.

That was one of the great things about living in the Shire, everywhere was within walking distance.

At 3.45 am, while Jane was fast asleep and snoring next to an empty tube of sour cream and onion Pringles, Debbie and I crept quietly out of Jane's back door, down the side of her house and onto the street. My pain had vanished and I was hoping it wouldn't come back at all.

'I can't believe we're doing this,' whispered Debbie. 'I can't wait to see Ashley and kiss him again. We should be jumping up and down, but we're already running late.'

'Do you want to run?' I asked.

'Yes,' replied Debbie and we sprinted all the way to Ashley's house.

We arrived outside, breathless and exhilarated, and flopped onto the gutter. Once we had caught our breaths, we crouched down behind a car in the street. We listened, holding on to each other, and occasionally popped our heads up from behind the car to try to see down Ashley's long dark driveway.

Then we saw someone walking towards us along the driveway, but it was so dark it could've been anyone. We both got ready to sprint away.

'Who is it?' Debbie hissed.

'It's a guy,' I said. 'It looks like a guy with long, shoulder-length hair.'

'Is it Ashley?' whispered Deb hopefully.

'Debbie!' whispered the figure loudly. 'Debbie? Kirsty? Are you out here?'

Debbie stood up from our hiding spot. 'Yes, who's that?'

'It's Jake!'

I stood up too and Jake walked over to us. Then Geoff and Ben joined us.

'Where's Ashley?' demanded Debbie.

'Ahh … we couldn't keep him awake so we thought we'd cover him in clothes pegs instead,' Geoff explained.

Debbie punched Geoff in the arm.

We all lay down on our backs in the middle of the road and waited for the sun to begin to make its appearance. Jake was next to me.

'Do you have a photo of anyone inside that locket you're always wearing?' he asked.

'Yeah.' I clicked it open and showed him. 'It's my friend Melissa who died of cancer.'

'Oh, that's the friend you mentioned in your speech at the swim-a-thon?'

I nodded.

'I'm sorry.'

'It's okay. You didn't do anything wrong,' I said.

'You know, it's weird how that's what people say.'

'I think it's because it's so sad that we don't know what else to say. I think people mean they're sorry you've had something painful happen to you,' I explained.

'You have really beautiful hands.' As he said this, insects began crawling inside my belly. I clicked my locket shut and pretended I hadn't heard his compliment. We all continued to talk in hushed voices until we heard something ... footsteps on the gravel.

Debbie and I bolted back to our hiding spot and the boys sat up and waited to see who it was. We waited and waited ... and then, a voice spoke ...

'You sneaky little buggers!'

Standing over us in her blue dressing gown and pink slippers was Ashley's mum.

We knew that we weren't in any real trouble, because Ashley's mum was pretty cool, but we were aware that we'd forced her out of bed at four-thirty in the morning and no mother would appreciate that.

'Sorry, Mrs Johnson,' we said in unison.

'I can't believe you two girls,' said Mrs Johnson. 'Kirsty, I thought you were a good young lady who performs in the theatre and does charity work. And Debbie, what would your father say? Now, boys, get back inside and girls, you'd better go home.'

Debbie and I waved goodbye to the boys and began walking back to Jane's place. As we turned our backs on Ashley's house, we heard Mrs Johnson mutter one more time: 'You sneaky little buggers!'

CHAPTER 20

Pain Haze

Medical waiting rooms are all the same. Sure, sometimes there are minor differences — maybe there's a sad-looking fish tank in the corner or a cheap poster on the wall — but in essence and atmosphere, they're the same. All the waiting rooms I've ever been in contain uncomfortable chairs that force you to sit up in an unnaturally straight-backed position. There are always old copies of magazines, and a token children's corner with tattered toys that somebody donated thirty years ago. The carpet is always ugly and the decor depressing, despite someone's well-intentioned attempt to get the carpet and uncomfortable chairs to match. Strangers sit together listening to the faint sound of the radio and staring listlessly at the fish tank or the pictures on the wall — poor distractions from the reality that they're suspended in.

Waiting rooms are worse than treatment rooms or doctors' rooms because all you can do in a waiting room is wait. You're in limbo. You have no power. I wonder how many hours of my life I've spent in waiting rooms. It would definitely be longer than the time I've actually spent with doctors. The key to surviving waiting rooms is to not let the room force you to wait. You need to find something to do so you forget that you're waiting. I read books. It works. I forget where I am and why I'm here, and fill my mind with people and places that have nothing to do with the medical world. Books are magic.

Today, I was having a lot of difficulty focusing on my book. I was here to find out my blood test results from my yearly check-up. My back pain hadn't come back and I was hoping it would stay that way.

Finally, after what felt like an eternity: 'Kirsty?'

'Come on, love,' said Mum, putting down the magazine she had been reading.

I left the waiting room, but I knew I would be back. I would always have to come back to get my blood checked. I sat down with Mum and yet another registrar I would never see again in the consultation room.

Here we go. Oh god ...

'Your blood count looks normal,' said the registrar.

'What?' I blurted out.

'Yep, everything is normal. Red blood cells and platelets are all good ...'

'What about my white blood cells?' Adrenaline made the tips of my fingers numb.

'Normal.'

Normal? How can that be?

'Were you expecting us to find something wrong?' asked the registrar.

'Maybe ... I've been getting really bad headaches and back pain that's so strong it feels like it's knocking the wind out of me.'

'She's also been looking very pale lately and she isn't eating much,' added Mum.

Have I been looking pale? Have I been eating less?

'Well, your blood count is completely normal,' said the registrar again. 'The headaches might be hormonal and the back pain ... I'm not sure about the back pain. It could be nerve damage — I can see here in your history you've had a lot of lumbar punctures. I'll write you a script for Panadeine Forte and that should take care of things. If that doesn't stop the pain, make sure you let us know. But there's nothing here in your blood results that worries me.'

So why do I still feel uneasy? I'm being silly. The results are right there and they're normal.

'All right, then,' said Mum. We got up to leave.

It's okay, I reassured myself. *You're okay. Blood can't lie. Can it?*

* * *

I ate an apple in front of Mum as soon as we got home from the hospital and asked her if Chris could come over for a swim.

'Of course, love. Is everything all right?'

'Yeah,' I lied. I swallowed two Panadeine Forte tablets with a glass of water and went to put on my bikini.

Dad had built our above-ground pool in the yard just before I was born. He kept it immaculately clean. The water was so clear you could see every tiny detail on the bottom of the pool. It never stank of chlorine, and every night Dad would check the chemical levels with a plastic kit that looked like a miniature chemistry set.

As I walked towards the pool, clutching my towel, I looked up at all the big trees surrounding the pool. Behind me were the massive wattles that our neighbour to the left of us had planted along their side of the fence. Mum hated them because she said the yellow flowers made her sneeze and attracted too many bees. Our other neighbours whose backyard met with ours had a huge tree that boasted enormous pink flowers. When we weren't home, the kids at that house would climb up that tree, jump over the fence and sneak into our pool. Down near our garage to my right were the trees Dad had planted — grevilleas with their sweet-tasting pods, and paperbarks. They were so small when Dad had put them in the ground, but now they were gigantic and looked like they'd always been there.

I sat on the edge of the pool and slunk my body into the water. It whooshed around me and swallowed me up so I was a part of it. I whipped my arms around just enough to keep me near the bottom. I could feel every single inch of my skin at the same time.

I think the Panadeine Forte is starting to work. I wonder if this is what the drug ecstasy feels like?

I lifted my legs behind me and positioned my feet against the wall of the pool. I stretched my hands in front of me and pushed off, pulling myself through the depths as hard as I could until my arms were right down by my sides. My body moved gracefully forwards. I let it rise. My face emerged up into the air and I opened my mouth and breathed in a deep lungful of oxygen.

Chris appeared. Mum must've let him in and told him where I was. He smiled at me as he pulled off his t-shirt, revealing his tanned lithe torso, and slipped into the water with me.

Words were squatting on my tongue like a toad. I let them out.

'Chris, I can't be your girlfriend. I just have this feeling in my stomach that I can't ignore. Do you understand? Have you ever had that feeling in your gut that's telling you to do something and you don't know why, you just know that you have to listen to it?'

'Yeah,' he said. 'The night I met you, my gut told me I had to kiss you and I had to have you.' His words made my heart hurt. 'Did everything go all right at your appointment? Is there something you're not telling me?'

'My appointment was fine.' I reached my tiny arms up towards his wide shoulders. 'I'm so sorry.'

He was an ice sculpture as soon as I touched him.

'Give me a proper hug,' I instructed him.

His rigid body melted and he leaned down, just like he always did, and hugged me back. I breathed in his scent of Lynx deodorant and saltwater. I gave him a final squeeze and let go. As I did, he caught my gaze. He was looking so hard into my eyes that I was worried he could read my thoughts. I suddenly felt like kissing him, but I didn't.

'You're so beautiful, Kirst.'

My soul soared. I pulled my eyes away.

'Promise me that we'll stay friends?' I asked. 'I mean it. I know lots of people just say that, but I mean it. I want us to be friends.'

He nodded.

We climbed out of the pool together and dried off. I walked him out and watched him get on his bike. He looked up, secured his helmet on his head and waved. He pushed off and began pedalling. I waved goodbye, even though he couldn't see me.

* * *

I was walking home along Hotham Road towards the Kingsway in Gymea, relieved it was the last day of school for 1997. My headache battered along with my footsteps, malevolently blurring my vision, forcing my eyes to squint and furrowing my brow. I was being kept company by my buddies — the big gumtrees that lined the footpath. It's almost impossible to walk down any street in the Shire without huge gumtrees swirling and swaying in the breeze and stretching up and up, dangerously close to the powerlines.

School had allowed us to ditch our uniforms so I was in my favourite t-shirt. It was white, and I'd made Mum get it for me because of the quote on it that read 'Sun, surf and smiles'. I lived in this t-shirt and I hated it when it was in the wash. I also had on a comfy pair of cargo shorts that I don't think had ever been washed. My black thongs beat the footpath as I passed Gymea TAFE. A group of mechanic students wolf-whistled at me and, as always, I ignored them.

I heard rapid footsteps behind me and I moved to the left side of the footpath to let the jogger run past me. I turned my head ever so slightly so they knew I was aware of their presence and letting them pass. But the footsteps stopped when they reached me and a familiar face grinned at me.

'Hey ... what are you doing coming along this way?' I asked.

'Umm ... I just wanted to ask you something ...' Jake stood in front of me, looking very gawky. He repeatedly shifted his school bag on his shoulder. 'Can I hug you?'

I need some Panadeine Forte.

'Sure,' I said.

I wrapped my small arms around his skinny waist and lifted my body up onto my toes. I could smell his long blond surfer-guy hair. It smelled a little bit like bleach and Rexona deodorant. Jake's sun-kissed arms hugged me in a delicate sort of way, like he thought if he hugged too hard that he might break me. He let go and placed both of his hands on my shoulders.

'Can I kiss you?' He breathed the words.

'Okay.'

What are you doing? You don't want a boyfriend. You want to get to the bottom of all this pain you're in and keep everyone else at a safe distance …

Very, very gently, Jake pushed his lips onto mine. He was handling me so softly, so carefully. His tongue lightly moved around the inside of my mouth. He held on to my head with his fingers tangled in my hair. My body began to buzz. When Chris kissed me, it was as if he liked me so much he was trying to consume me, but Jake was kissing me like I was a fragile fairy who might get wrecked if he didn't handle me with care.

'GET A ROOM!' one of the guys at the TAFE yelled out to us.

We stopped kissing.

'Can I walk you home?' Jake asked.

'Sure.'

He grabbed hold of my left hand and we floated along the footpath together. My lower spine had invisible fingers squeezing it. My headache continued to erratically bang around inside my skull.

'That's it, mate!' shouted the TAFE guy. 'Get her back to your place and finish what you started!'

CHAPTER 21

Unusual

It was school holidays and a sweltering summer, as it usually was in the Shire at that time of year. I spent a lot of my days hanging out with Debbie and our friends, and occasionally I would see Jake, but my body seemed to be running on erratic mode lately, especially at night-time, when my head would pound in pain and my lower back would relentlessly pulse and pierce shots of agony into me. Sleep became impossible. I kept taking Panadeine Forte, but it wasn't working. For a whole week, I barely slept. I would doze for a few minutes, and then shoot up in bed, gasping for air.

On the seventh night of torment, I woke up, bathed in sweat, and looked at the clock: 3.07 am. I threw the blue sheets off my bed and onto the floor. Pain drilled into my temples and my eyes felt like they were tennis balls, too large to fit in my head and covered in fuzz that made them gritty and itchy. For hours,

I stared at the blue ceiling and my blue dolphin wind chime, which Dad had hung up for me near my window. My abdomen began to spasm. I placed one hand on my tummy and clutched my locket in the other. Then, with melancholy weighing on my soul, I sat up and walked through to my parents' bedroom.

'Mum?' I said into the darkness. 'Dad?'

They both sat up.

'What is it?' asked Mum.

'You need to take me to the hospital. The pain ... the pain has become so bad and the Panadeine isn't helping. We need to go now.'

'All right, love,' she answered.

My parents fumbled around in the dark.

'We need to go to the hospital at Randwick,' I said, leaning against the door frame. 'Something feels wrong.'

Mum and Dad froze when they heard my request to go to Randwick instead of the local hospital. Randwick was the 'cancer hospital'. The place I'd been free of for over four years. The place you only went to when something was horribly wrong.

* * *

The hospital at Randwick wasn't Prince of Wales Children's Hospital any more; it was now Sydney Children's Hospital. It was no longer a dismal poo-coloured place, but a modern, yellow and very cheerful-looking building.

I lay on the firm hospital bed in the early morning daylight, feeling defeated. I knew what was coming. I was certainly not okay with it, but I was trying to stay calm.

Dr Sue Russell came into the room. She had replaced the Prof, who'd retired, but he still pottered around in the realm of his cancer kids. He continued to see some patients who were off treatment and in remission, and he was still involved in the Children's Cancer Institute of Australia, which would not have come into existence without him. Dr Sue had brown, wild, shoulder-length hair that contained little flickers of grey. She was in her early forties and her clothes looked like they either hadn't been ironed, or she'd slept in them. She didn't wear any make-up and seemed frazzled.

She studied my chart for a few moments and said, 'I really don't think your leukaemia has come back, Kirsty. Your blood results look normal, but just to be absolutely certain we'll do a lumbar puncture and bone marrow biopsy. We'll give you some happy gas to make it a little more comfortable for you.'

'Okay,' I said, slightly relieved that I wouldn't have to endure the needles cold turkey like I used to.

'Do you want someone to come with you?' said Dr Sue.

I looked at Mum and Dad. Mum's skin had turned grey and, to my alarm, Dad looked frail. My vibrant and healthy father, who surfed almost every day, looked like he was having trouble standing up.

I don't want to put Mum and Dad through this again. They don't need to see me have any more lumbar punctures and bone marrow biopsies. They've seen enough horror because of me. Am I destined to be the child in the family that causes everyone else to be worried all the time?

'I'll go in by myself,' I said to Dr Sue.

'Are you sure, love?' asked Mum, but I could already see relief wash over her. I can't say I blamed her. Who on earth would want to see anyone have these tests done?

'Yep, I'm sure,' I said.

Dad seemed to wobble, but he managed to stay upright. He had the strangest look on his face. What was this bizarre expression that had deformed Dad's features?

Oh my gosh, Dad is scared. This is awful. I don't want to be the reason why Dad has this look.

'Walk around to the treatment room,' said Dr Sue. 'They're ready for you. I'll come and see you later on. I really don't think it's your leukaemia. You've been in remission for over four years. It's very unlikely that it would come back now.'

I pushed the stiff white hospital sheet off my legs and got off the bed. I was wearing my favourite boxer shorts. They were blue-and-white striped silk, covered in Bananas in Pyjamas. I also had on my favourite t-shirt, the 'Sun, surf and smiles' one I was wearing when Jake kissed me. On my own, I walked around to the left past the nurses' station and into the treatment room.

The treatment room was the whitest, coldest and most intimidating room I'd ever been in. It was fully equipped for any doctor to walk in and perform surgery. Goose bumps erupted all over my skin and my breathing became shallow. I wondered if doctors had become any better at performing lumbar punctures.

'You can hop up when you're ready,' someone said.

A flat table that looked like a thickly padded ironing board loomed large in front of me. It was covered in a plastic sheet, and when I placed my feet on the small step and then perched my body on the edge of the table, the plastic stuck to the backs of my legs.

'Whenever you're ready, just lie down on your side and curl up for us,' someone else instructed me.

I nodded like an obedient, emotionless robot. I lay on my side with my back to the voices and curled up as tight as I could into a ball. All I could see was a bright white wall. I pulled my knees up under my chin even closer and tighter, then someone placed a rubber gas mask over my nose and mouth.

'Just take some long deep breaths,' I was told.

The smell of the gas was strong. It was metallic and sickly at first, but the more I breathed it in, the less I seemed to notice how rank it was. My thoughts became scrambled and the world started to blur.

This feels so trippy. Am I dreaming this? Maybe this isn't real.

I felt a cold splash of antiseptic on my back and the piercing deep sting of the needle as it entered my lower spine, but these things were only vaguely in my awareness. The gas made me feel like I sort of didn't mind, or didn't care, that I was enduring this awful procedure yet again.

Am I really here? Who am I? My eyes feel heavy. I'm so tired. I think I'll just go to sleep. Ouch … something is stinging my back. I'm having a test or something, aren't I? I can't focus. Why can't I focus? I don't like this, but I can't be bothered to do anything.

* * *

The gas must have put me to sleep. I woke up back in bed, glad not to be in the blinding treatment room. Dr Sue was standing near my feet. She seemed to look at me for a long time, or maybe I was still a bit trippy from the gas. I tried to push myself up. My lower back and my hip felt stingy and achy. My hair felt itchy and greasy. When was the last time I'd washed it?

'Kirsty,' said Dr Sue after what felt like a long while, 'I'm really sorry. Your blood was showing up as normal, but when we looked at the spinal fluid … Your leukaemia has come back.'

I didn't cry. I didn't scream. I didn't even move. One word came to mind.

'Shit,' I breathed out.

'We need to get a central line put into you. Your veins aren't in very good shape from the first time you were treated and we need to get some chemo into you as soon as we can.'

Melissa had a central line. Melissa died. Oh Melissa ... what's going to happen to me?

'I'll get someone to come and explain how the central line works,' Dr Sue continued. 'We'll need to be careful where we put it, so you can still wear a bra. You'll need to be here for at least a few weeks.'

I nodded mutely.

'We'll also look into getting you a bone marrow transplant, which is your best chance at survival. But we need to find someone who's a match for you first.'

I slowly nodded again.

'And, Kirsty,' said Dr Sue, 'I am really sorry about this. I didn't think your cancer would come back again. It's quite unusual for someone to relapse this late.'

Unusual? Oh geez — who on earth would ever want their doctor to refer to them as 'unusual'?

I sat there, very still.

'We'll need to move you to the ward,' said Dr Sue. She didn't say 'cancer ward' because she knew that I knew exactly what she meant. 'You're sixteen years old now, so if you want to go over to the adult hospital you can, but we're happy to have you here. It's entirely up to you.'

'I'll stay in the Children's Hospital,' I said.

'I think that's a good idea,' Dr Sue said. 'I'll come to see you again tomorrow.'

Dr Sue left me with Mum and Dad. Without a word, Dad gave me a hug and went home.

It was 18 January 1998 and I had cancer for the second time.

'Do you want to call Danielle?' asked Mum.

I nodded.

Mum rang Danielle and broke the news about my diagnosis. Then she handed me the phone.

'Hey sis.' As soon as I heard Danielle's voice, I felt less overwhelmed. 'Is there anything you want or need me to do for you?'

'Actually, there is,' I said. 'I'm going to give you a list of people and I need you to call them and tell them I've got cancer again. Make sure you tell them that I'm going to be fine. I know it's probably going to freak people out, but tell them not to worry about me, okay?'

'Okay, Kirst.'

'Mum will bring the list home to you.'

'All right. What did the doctor say?'

'She said I've got to have a central line put in and start some chemo before I get to come home. It's going to be a few weeks.' I didn't even sound like me. My voice was flat, a warped variation of what I usually sounded like.

Mum started waving at me to get off the phone so she could speak to Danielle again. I handed it to her and lay back in the rigid hospital bed, listening to Mum telling Danielle to put on a couple of loads of washing.

CHAPTER 22

My Favourite Roommate

'Is it okay if Kirsty shares a room with you, Matthew?'

Fragile, flat and barely able to hold my body up, I patiently waited to see if I would be granted entry into a hospital room with only one other patient in it. This was a very big deal. Privacy is a privilege that's as slippery as soap to grasp onto when you stay in hospital. I smiled at the patient. He looked about six or seven years old, but when children are bald and stricken with cancer it's trickier to guess our ages. His eyes, which had dark grey smudges under them, were huge and they pierced right into my core as he scanned my face and then my body. He'd obviously had this room to himself for some time, so I can't say I'd have blamed him if he told me to 'nick off'.

I decided to speak up. Maybe I could help him to make up his mind.

'I have a little brother called Matthew,' I said.

He didn't respond.

'He's my favourite brother,' I continued, clinging on to my IV pole. Suddenly I had his attention.

'You're not supposed to have favourite brothers,' he informed me.

'Yeah, I know,' I said, 'but my little brother likes all the same things that I do, like movies and food, and he makes me laugh.'

At this moment, Matthew's mother, a gorgeous lioness of a woman with a stunning, thick, curly mane of brown hair, joined our conversation. 'Matthew, do you think you'd like to share a room with Kirsty for a while?' She winked at me as she said this and I smiled at her, shifting back and forth on my anaemic and unsteady legs.

'What is your little brother's favourite food?' he asked me.

'Well, he likes all sorts of stuff, like McDonald's and pizza and Chinese food ...' I said.

'Do you and your brother like KFC?'

I could tell this was a test. This would be the decider as to whether this little boy with cancer would let me share his room. Maybe he hated KFC. Maybe he loved it. Judging by the way his face lit up when he asked the question, I made an educated guess.

'Yeah, we like KFC,' I said, injecting enthusiasm into my voice.

'All right, you can stay in here with me,' he said. 'I'm having KFC for dinner tonight. Do you want to have some with me? My mum is going to get it for me. She can get some for you too.'

'I'd love some,' I said.

A smirk ignited upon his face.

I pushed my IV pole towards the bed that was opposite my new KFC-loving friend. Mum trailed behind me, plonked my things near the bed that would be my home for at least a few weeks and pulled back the nasty rigid sheets. I plugged my IV into the power point in the wall and climbed into bed, but I didn't lie down.

Mum went over and introduced herself to Matthew's mum. This ritual is an important one. Children and parents on cancer wards are inevitably going to be spending a lot of time together, so setting up a positive relationship can help make your stay a little bit more bearable. Ask me 'What's the worst thing about cancer?', and my answer is 'People.' Ask me 'What's the best thing about cancer?', and my answer is 'People.' We have the capacity to make life better and we also have the capacity to make life worse. We have all the power — it's up to us how we choose to use it.

While Matthew's mum was getting us takeaway, I got Mum to set up a chair next to his bed so we could eat together.

The smell of KFC was overwhelming when she returned. Saliva flooded my mouth. Together, our mums set up a little bed picnic. They wheeled over a small table and unpacked the food for us. The red-and-white striped boxes of chicken and chips with their tasty chicken salt were popped open, releasing a cloud of steam and the strong smell of oily potato.

Matthew grabbed a drumstick in his fist and bit into it, making noises of pleasure like it was the best thing he had ever eaten. I grabbed a breast and picked off small pieces of skin. It was greasy and salty and so good. I hadn't had solid food for so long that my body was a bit shocked by the sensations of eating.

'KFC have the best chips ever,' Matthew told me, before shoving three into his mouth at the same time. 'It's the special salt they use.'

I grinned at him and took a chip and sucked on it, letting it dissolve in my mouth.

The chicken quickly disappeared. Matthew ate far more of it than I did. We tore open the lemon-scented moist towelettes and wiped our hands. We had just experienced a sort of sensory ecstasy. The smell of the chicken and the heavily salted chips, and the feel of the grease running down our fingers and chins, had been divine. I wondered if having an unhealthy body made unhealthy food taste better. Or maybe it was Matthew's joy at the simple pleasure of food rubbing off on me. For at least ten minutes, my new friend and I had been eating like little piggies, abandoning the reality of where we were and loving every second of it.

When we finished and our mums had thrown away the chicken bones and boxes, a sadness fell over me. This blissful and comforting experience was over, and now I would have to go back to bed and swallow forty tablets. As I stood up and placed my hand on my IV pole, I smiled at my new roommate and said, 'Thanks for the KFC. That was so good.'

'It's the best,' he said. He put his hand on his tummy. 'I'm so full.'

'Me too,' I said. 'I'll have dinner with you any time you want, okay?'

'Yeah,' he said and smiled widely.

Suddenly, his smile vanished. Standing in the doorway was his oncologist. I pushed my IV pole back over to my own bed and climbed in.

'Hello, Matthew, how are you feeling this evening?' said his doctor.

'Good,' he said. 'I had KFC for dinner with Kirsty.'

'Did you save any for me?'

'No!' he replied, as if this was a ridiculous question.

'Oh well, maybe next time then,' said his doctor. 'I just wanted to come around and let you know that it looks like we'll probably be able to send you home in a few days. How do you feel about that?'

'Really?' Matthew was astonished.

'I think so, as long as nothing changes and you keep feeling all right.'

'Oh, thank you,' gushed Matthew's mum. 'That's great news.'

'All right, well, I'll see you again tomorrow,' said the doctor. 'Goodnight, Matthew.'

The doctor left and Matthew's mum pulled her son into her chest, hugging him tightly. She picked up the phone by his bed and started calling a bunch of people to tell them the good news.

Then I had a visit from Dr Sue. She was already giving me chemotherapy intravenously, but there were still lots of things to sort out, like getting a central line and trying to find a bone marrow match so I could have a transplant. 'Hi, Kirsty,' she said. 'How are you feeling?'

'I have a headache and my back hurts, but I'm all right. You don't know when I'll be able to go home yet, do you?'

'I can't really answer that for you at this stage. Has someone explained to you about the central line yet?'

'No,' I said.

The only thing I know about central lines is that Melissa had one.

'I'll make sure someone tells you about it. We also need to test your brothers and sister as soon as possible; hopefully one of them will be a match for you so we can give you a bone marrow transplant. We'll check the Bone Marrow Registry as well to see if there's a stranger who's a match. I really think a transplant is the best way to go.'

I nodded, but a question nagged at the back of my mind.

What if there's no match?

CHAPTER 23

Love Flood

'You know, everyone loves walking past your room, Kirsty,' said a nurse called Scott, as he took my blood pressure and temperature.

'How come?' I asked.

'The flowers. There's so many flowers in here that you can smell them out in the hall when you walk past. You must have a lot of people who care about you.'

My room was flooded with bouquets of flowers, 'Get Well Soon' balloons and cards, and teddy bears, and there was a steady stream of phone calls from all sorts of people wanting to pass on some positivity.

'Another bouquet of flowers just arrived, but I'm still trying to find a vase. I might need to borrow one from another ward.' Scott wrote down my blood pressure and temperature. They must've been okay because if they weren't, he would've told me.

A few minutes later, he returned with the most enormous bouquet of red roses I'd ever seen. 'It looks like someone loves you,' he commented cheekily.

'Was there a card?'

'No, just the flowers.'

Puzzlement planted itself on my face.

'So, I take it you've got a few admirers then.' He laughed as he made room for the roses among all the other bunches.

I blushed.

'I'm not surprised. A pretty, young girl like you ... if I was a sixteen-year-old boy, I'd ask you out.' Mischief twinkled in his eyes.

My cheeks flushed scarlet again and I rolled my eyes. Scott was an interesting-looking man, but not exactly my type. He had dark slicked-back hair that was neatly pulled into a ponytail at the base of his neck, and a goatee and moustache — kind of like one of the Three Musketeers. He had a silver nose ring that reminded me of the rings you often see in the nostrils of bulls, and silver and black piercings filled both of his ears.

Scott grinned and strolled out of the room.

Within moments, he'd returned again. 'There's a phone call on hold for you. Do you want to take it?' he asked.

'Who is it?'

'A very polite young gentleman who goes by the name of Chris.'

My heart went *plonk*.

'You should talk to him, love,' encouraged Mum from her chair in the corner.

I can't.

'Can you tell him I'm asleep or too sick to take calls or something?' I asked Scott.

'Are you sure?' Mum asked.

'Yeah, are you sure?' chimed Scott.

'Yes,' I said.

Scott hurried out. I stared at the stunning and what must've been extremely expensive long-stemmed red roses. I'd never been given roses by anyone before.

Scott returned. 'Chris wanted me to give you a message.' I nodded for him to go on. 'He wanted to check that you got the roses he sent and he wanted you to know that you can call him any time you feel up to it and that he's thinking of you.'

I stared at my white legs stretched out on the bed.

'That's very nice of him,' said Mum.

'Yep, he sounded very nice on the phone,' he added.

'I know,' I said quietly. 'Chris *is* very nice.'

And that's exactly why I want to keep him as far away from me and all this cancer crap as possible. If I speak to him, I might accidentally tell him the real reason I dumped him was because I had a feeling I was getting sick and I wanted to spare him all of the horrors that come with tumbling down the cancer tunnel.

'Maybe you'll feel up to calling him when you get home,' suggested Mum.

'Maybe ... I don't know.' And I really didn't.

* * *

Sundays are special on the oncology ward. You usually won't have any intense intravenous chemo, as there are not many doctors around if anything goes wrong. There's also a lady called Patsy, who works at the hospital and comes and cooks a barbecue for us kids and our families and visitors, only charging five dollars for a huge plate of homemade pastas and salads, as well as fresh fruit, sausages and steak. If you've ever had suspicions that there are angels masquerading as people among us humans, then Patsy would make you a believer for sure. But the most special thing of all about Sundays is that visitors can come pretty much all day.

For a few weeks, it had just been me and Mum, but my blood counts were finally good enough for me to have visitors. Mum got up early so she could use the one shower available to parents immediately after it had received its once-a-day cleaning. Then she took me to have a bath — I was too weak to stand up in a shower. We both washed and blow-dried our hair. We applied moisturiser to our whole bodies, blasted our armpits with deodorant and put on clean clothes. I usually just sat around in boxer shorts and a t-shirt, but today I put on shorts, wore a bra, and filed and shaped my nails. By the time I'd finished getting ready, I was exhausted. In my excitement to see people outside cancer-town, I'd forgotten I was a resident and that fatigue could make my body flop without warning. Mum made a wall of pillows on my bed to prop me up. I didn't want to greet any of my visitors lying down.

First, Dad arrived with Matt and Brett. My brothers both hugged me. I couldn't remember either of them hugging me before. Maybe Dad had told them to.

Dad gave me one of his patented hugs. Then he gave me one of the most valuable gifts you can give someone with cancer: a Discman. He also brought about twenty spare batteries, headphones and a huge pile of CDs for me to listen to: Phil Collins, The Beatles, The Carpenters, Abba, Midnight Oil ...

Had Brett and Matt become more handsome since I'd seen them last? I'd never thought of Brett as good-looking, but his copper mane of hair shone beautifully under the fluorescent hospital lights. Matt's Nutella-coloured skin appeared more perfect than ever before, and his dimples seemed more prominent. Brett handed me a stack of cards and letters addressed to me that had been delivered to the house. I pointed him towards the small fridge in my room. Every hospital meal on the kids' cancer ward came with a carton of chocolate or strawberry milk, and I'd been saving them all for Brett and Matt, who loved flavoured milk, but were never allowed to have it at home. They were both very grateful for this gift, and were kind enough not to mention that my relapse had led to a relaxation of this rule.

After more unexpected hugs from my brothers and another hug from Dad, it was time for them to go. Dr Sue had advised that any visitor should only stay for ten to thirty minutes, otherwise it would wear me out. As Dad gave me one last hug goodbye, he whispered, 'If you can't sleep, or you feel sick, or you're in pain, or you feel sad or scared or angry — or even if you feel all these things at once — I want you to promise me you'll just listen to some music, okay?'

'I promise,' I said. I felt as if he would've hugged me forever if I hadn't let go of him. My dad was so smart, he was already aware of what people now call 'music therapy'.

It wasn't long before the next shift of visitors arrived — Debbie and Geoff. Geoff brought me a 'Get Well Soon' card with small messages of kindness from him and his whole family. Debbie wrote me a poem that was covered in drawings of stars and the moon. She also brought me the latest copies of *Cleo*, *Cosmopolitan*, *Girlfriend* and *Dolly* magazines.

Then came my theatre friends — even the directors. They brought me teddy bears and lollies and one of the directors, my favourite one, Lyn, brought me videos of all the performances I'd ever been in over the last four years. Lyn always made a point of filming our performances and filing the videos away for safekeeping, but I'd never seen them before.

My final visitors for the day were Danielle, Jane and Jake. As I hugged Danielle, I whispered, 'I've gotta talk to Jake alone. Can you and Jane keep Mum occupied for a few minutes?'

Of course, any wish I made to Danielle was granted. She convinced Mum to go for a walk and get some fresh air. Jane chimed in, saying she'd buy them McDonald's.

I was alone with Jake.

My skin felt prickly and hot. Jake held my hand in between both of his sun-tanned hands.

'Jake, I can't be your girlfriend,' I said. 'I can't be anyone's girlfriend now that this has happened.'

'Shut up,' he said in a manner of joking gentleness.

'No. You need to listen to me. I'm really sick. I'm going to lose all of my hair. I won't even look like me any more. I think it's best if you just be my friend and not my boyfriend.'

'I told you to shut up,' he said. 'I'm not going to break up with you because you have cancer.'

'You don't have to. I'm breaking up with you.'

'Stop it, Kirst.'

'No. You have no idea how bad this is going to get.'

'Yeah, I do. A nurse came to school and explained everything to all of us.'

'You can't possibly understand. You need to trust me. You won't want to be my boyfriend and I don't need a boyfriend anyway. I just need you to be a friend.'

'You have plenty of friends already. Close your eyes and hold out your hands. I've got something for you. I didn't have any money to buy you expensive flowers so … I had to improvise.'

Reluctantly, I closed my eyes and held out my hands.

'Open your eyes.'

He'd handed me an exercise book that was covered in photographs of all our friends and in big capital letters he'd written the words, 'WE LUV YOU'.

'What is this?' I asked.

'Open it.'

I did as he said and on the first page the words 'AND I DO TOO' were written with a big red heart around them. My heart filled with glee.

Jake loves me?! Oh my goodness!

There was also a note:

Dear Kirsty,

I've never known someone who is so gorgeous, determined and gutsy. I've never known anyone with more heart than you. The pain this world puts us through is unfair, but always remember you've got a LOT of people who love you very much and I am one of them. I think about you 24hrs a day and will ALWAYS be here for you. All my love, Jakey. Oxoxox

'Keep turning the pages,' he instructed. The rest of the book was filled with notes from our friends and even students in our grade who weren't my close friends. He'd got as many people as he could to fill the pages with words of support and love. There were also photos, drawings and poems.

My face began to feel hot, as if I'd been severely sunburned. I began to feel woozy and lay down on my side.

'Thank you,' I said. 'It's such a nice thing ... I can't believe you did all of this for me.'

'I love you and I'm going to be there for you through this whole transplant thing.'

'Jake, no ... you don't understand.'

'Stop,' he insisted. 'Stop trying to push me away. I can handle this.'

No, you can't.

Mum, Danielle and Jane returned.

'What's wrong, love?' said Mum. 'Why are you lying down? Your face has blotches all over it.'

'I don't know what happened. We were just sitting here talking and then my face ... my face feels like it's on fire.'

'I think that's enough visiting for today,' said Mum sternly. 'I think it's best if the three of you get going.'

I lifted my hands to cover my face, but Jake gently grabbed my wrists. 'Remember what I said.'

All I could manage was a nod.

Danielle and Jane both gave me a quick goodbye kiss on the forehead. They left just before my face exploded in a rash of red blotches and bubbly pimples. I closed my eyes. I heard the nurse tell Mum it was a reaction to the steroids.

* * *

For the next couple of weeks, Jake called me every day as soon as he got home from school. Every time he did, I tried to break up with him, and every time he told me to 'shut up'. He delivered trinkets to me, like mini teddy bears, mix tapes he'd made for me, bouquets of flowers he'd picked from the gardens in his street, countless love letters, hand–drawn pictures and funny short stories he wrote himself.

Was it possible for a sixteen-year-old boy to want a girlfriend with cancer?

CHAPTER 24

A New Gown

It was the morning that my central line was to be inserted in my body. I was minutes away from being wheeled into surgery when a nurse *finally* came to explain things to me.

'Central lines are great,' she said. She had the husky voice of a smoker and she smelled like cigarettes and cheap perfume. 'You're used to having people trying to put cannulas into a vein every time you have to have chemotherapy, or a blood test, or a blood or platelet transfusion, but with a central line, we just unscrew the cap and hook you up to your IV or take blood or inject chemo.'

'So … it won't hurt when I have IV treatments?' I asked. This seemed a little too good to be true.

'Nope, you won't have to endure needles in the skin any more. The central line is just a tube that will be connected to a vein near your heart inside your body. The surgeon will cut open the skin near your collarbone and insert the tube. You'll see it coming out of your chest just here' — she tapped on the flesh that was just above my right breast — 'and where it comes out it splits into two tubes, so we can give you chemo and a transfusion of blood at the same time.'

'All right …' I said.

So I won't have to put up with registrars who can't find veins? This may not be so bad.

'Oh, and you can't get a central line wet, so that means you won't be able to have showers or go swimming.' She said this to me like it was not a big deal at all.

'What?'

'You can't get it wet or it can get infected. If it gets water or soap in it, or if you go into a pool or the ocean, it increases your chances of getting an infection and, well … cancer patients can die from central line infections.'

'How am I supposed to wash?'

'Most patients just have baths with a little bit of water in them. Like a bird bath, you know. A wardsman is going to take you into surgery in a minute. I've just got to find him.'

I can do this. It will be okay. Melissa was younger than me and she could handle having a central line, so I need to suck it up.

The wardsman arrived to wheel me into surgery to collect my body's new accessory. Matthew waved from his hospital bed as I went past him, and I waved back.

* * *

'Kirsty? Kirsty? Can you try to open your eyes for us, sweetie?'

A kind woman's voice was trying to pull me out of the heavy veil of anaesthetic. I tried to open my eyes, but they felt like they were taped shut.

'Kirsty, can you squeeze my finger and try to open your eyes?' A cold finger placed itself inside my hand. I willed myself as hard as I could to fight the leftover druggy feeling from the anaesthetic. Weakly, I squeezed her finger.

'Good, good job. Now do you think you could try opening your eyes for me?'

I am trying.

'Are you in any pain?' the kind voice asked. As soon as she mentioned it, the pain came to life.

Oh my god! My neck!

My right collarbone screamed with a wasp-sting-like pain that I'd never experienced before. It felt like someone was taking a sharp scalpel to my collarbone and slicing me open as I lay there.

Have I woken up in surgery? I've heard that can happen ... oh my gosh, it hurts so badly.

My eyes began to water from the dreadful stinging sensation. With my eyes still shut, I opened my mouth ever so slightly and said, 'Is it done? Is the central line put in? Is the surgery over?'

'Yes, Kirsty. It's all over and it went well. You're in recovery now. We'll wheel you back to the ward, but we just need you to try to open your eyes for us first, okay?'

Why is it so hard to just open my eyes?

'Kirsty, just try and open your eyes for a second or two, and then you can go back to sleep, all right?'

Come on, Kirst. Just open your eyes. Easy peasy. Come on.

I forced my lids to open a millimetre or two. Bright light shone into the tiny slits.

'Just a bit more, Kirsty ...'

I forced them wider. More tears ran down my cheeks as the light blinded me. The pain in my collarbone was brutal. It felt like they hadn't sewn up the wound yet, though I knew they must have.

'That's it!' The nurse with the kind voice seemed ecstatic. 'All right, we'll take you back to the ward now so you can rest.'

* * *

As soon as I was back in my room, I realised that I needed to pee really badly. I guessed I'd have to open my eyes so I could get to the bathroom.

'I really need to go to the bathroom,' I said to the nurse on the ward who was getting me settled. I was busting to the point that it was starting to hurt my abdomen.

'I'll go get you a bedpan,' said the nurse.

'No,' I said. 'I'm not peeing in a bedpan. My mum can walk me to the bathroom.'

'It's not a good idea, Kirsty,' she said. 'You've only just woken up from surgery. I'll just quickly run and get you a bedpan.' She went to leave.

'Wait,' said Mum. 'Kirsty doesn't use bedpans.'

I forced my eyes open in determination. My stinging collarbone pulsated as I lifted the paper-like sheets off my legs and used my elbows to push myself up. I wanted some dignity. I did not want to sit on my bed, on a bedpan, with just the flimsy 'privacy curtain' drawn and my new friend Matthew listening. No way. I swung my legs over the side of the bed.

'Kirsty, love,' said Mum, 'it may not be a good idea. We don't want you to fall over or anything.'

'Mum, I'm going to walk to the bathroom to pee. I'd like you to help me, but if you don't, I'll just take myself.'

'All right, love,' said Mum. She came around to help me stand. 'Let's walk really slowly. Take your time.'

I shuffled, not even lifting my feet off the ground, and every step closer to that bathroom made me feel like I'd done the right thing. Eventually, we reached the door.

'Should I come in with you?' Mum asked.

'No, Mum. I can pee on my own,' I said.

'All right, well, I'm going to wait right outside this door, so don't lock it from the inside. The buzzer is right next to the toilet, so if you start feeling dizzy, press it and yell out and I'll come in.'

I lifted the white hospital gown, causing a sharp pain in my neck and collarbone, then pulled my knickers down and sat on the toilet. My feet did not touch the floor, so I reached out my hand and grabbed the cold metal railing on the wall to stabilise myself. As the peeing came to an end, a small ripple of relief shook through my body. I had a wee orgasm. You know what I mean; I know you do. When you're busting and you finally get to go. *Ahh!*

I wiped myself with the cheap scratchy toilet paper that hospitals are always stocked with, pulled my knickers back up, and dropped the gown back down. I was about to stand when I looked up and saw myself in a full-length mirror that was absurdly positioned in front of the toilet. I sucked in a breath as I looked at my reflection.

Is that me?

I began to shuffle closer to the mirror. I wasn't bald yet, but my hair was filthy and hung lifelessly around my oily face.

Argh ... I look dreadful. I need to get someone to wash my hair. I'll be bald soon, but I want my hair to look clean while I still have it.

I washed my hands with lots of soap, dried them with paper towels, then soaked some of the paper towels with water and wiped the oil off my face. My skin was deathly white and my once-toned legs were wasted and skinny. In the oversized hospital gown, my body looked tiny.

I want to have a look at this central line.

Mum knocked loudly on the door. 'Are you all right in there, Kirsty?'

'Yeah, Mum! I'm just washing my hands. I'll be out in a second!'

'All right, love. Take your time. Don't rush.'

I took a deep breath and lifted my hospital gown, up over my flat tummy; up over my tiny boobs, which seemed even tinier than ever; and then up onto my shoulders, revealing the central line to me.

Oh my …

Protruding from my chest was a tube that divided into two white tubes, both about fifteen centimetres long. Where the tube exited my body, they had stuck a clear square of plastic to protect the wound from germs. At the end of the two tubes were little plastic clamps and small caps that they could unscrew to hook me up to intravenous treatment. They were just like the caps on Melissa's central line. It was a huge monstrosity. I was now sentenced to loose-fitting tops only, unless I wanted people to see this beast. Disgusted at the sight, I dropped the hospital gown, turned on the taps and splashed water on my face.

I've got an alien squatting half inside my body and half outside. No one warned me it would be like this. They said it would make everything easier.

Suddenly, a sensation began to build and spread from the square of plastic on my chest. Sweat began to gather above my eyebrows and on my upper lip. A red circle appeared on my hospital gown. It began to grow bigger. My head felt groggy as this patch of blood grew and spread down the front of my body. As it spread, it turned from warm to cold and I began to shiver. The starched white hospital gown was becoming a red dress. A gown of blood.

'Mum!' I yelled out.

Mum burst through the door. 'Oh my god, you've split open the stitches.'

People came rushing into the bathroom and all I could think was, *I didn't know my teeny thirty-nine-kilogram body would have so much blood in it.*

CHAPTER 25

Tantrum

I could tell by the sunlight streaming into the room that it was the afternoon when I woke. But it was not the dazzling sun that had woken me — it was the voice of Matthew's oncologist.

'I'm very sorry, Matthew, but I don't think we'll be able to let you go home tomorrow. Your blood counts don't look very good. Maybe in a week or so, we'll see if we can get you home.'

There was only silence.

The doctor said nothing more and left.

Mum went over to Matthew's mum and put her arm around her shoulders. 'Do you want to go for a walk and get a cup of coffee?' she asked.

Unable to speak in her devastation, Matthew's mum nodded.

'Kirsty will keep an eye on Matthew,' said Mum.

I gave a small nod, but it hurt my neck. My body wasn't used to having a tube inside it yet. The pain in my collarbone meant it was agonising to turn my head or look up or down.

Mum came over and grabbed her purse and sunglasses. 'We'll be back in a bit,' she whispered to me. 'Matthew is probably too weak to get out of bed and you need to lie still so you don't pop open your stitches again.' I playfully rolled my eyes at her. 'See you soon.'

I moved my eyes so I could see Matthew. He had his arms folded across his chest and I could hear him breathing heavily, like he was trying to not explode with anger. I can't say I blamed him. The possibility of going home is what keeps you sane in here and someone had just taken this away from him. He should've been going to school, playing soccer with his friends and enjoying just being a kid, but fate had arranged alternative plans. I wanted to say something to make him feel better, but what could I possibly say? I'd been in this situation many times before and there was nothing that anyone could say that would make me feel better. So I said nothing.

He was fuming now and I imagined steam blasting out of his ears. *Let him be as angry as he pleases*, I thought. I watched him look around frantically. His eyes landed on a few plastic cups on a table next to his bed. They had once been filled with tablets, but now they were empty. He threw each cup onto the floor, one after the other. Tears filled his eyes as he ran out of cups.

I had a pile of the same cups next to me. I scooped them up in my hands. The stack was like a long snake made out of Lego pieces. I launched the snake towards his bed and it landed near his feet. One at a time, he slammed my collection of cups in all directions, so the floor looked like it was covered in plastic-cup confetti. If he wasn't attached to an IV pole, I'm sure he would've stormed out of the ward. He should've been able to if he wanted, but even his fury was stifled by this place.

I finally dared to speak. 'Matthew.'

'I wanna go home! It's not fair!'

'I know. I wanna go home too. One day, when we don't have to come to this place any more, we should go and eat KFC in the restaurant.'

He was so furious I couldn't even cheer him up with his favourite topic.

'It would make me really happy to eat KFC with you when we're not in hospital. Can you promise me we'll do it one day? You can be my date.'

'You're too old for me,' he said.

'Yeah, I know. We can just go as friends then. Do you promise me?'

'I promise,' he replied.

Scott came into the room. Immediately, he noticed all the cups on the floor, but he didn't react to them. He knew Matthew had just received the bad news that he'd be staying at Hotel Cancer a little longer.

'Hey Matthew, do you like *Star Wars*?' he asked.

'Yes,' Matthew answered with a snap.

'I've got an idea. I'll be right back.'

Ten minutes later Scott returned, pushing a metal trolley that had all sorts of hospital supplies on it. There were piles of plastic kidney-shaped bowls that patients used to vomit in sometimes. There were empty syringes with no needles, cardboard toilet rolls, bandages, bedpans, straws and foam cups. 'Wanna build a space station?'

Matthew's rage went from boiling point to a low simmer. 'Yeah! I have a better idea for how the Death Star should've been built.'

'Let's do it,' said Scott and, under Matthew's careful instruction, they built a space station out of hospital supplies. When they'd finished, Scott found some string and hung it from the ceiling right above Matthew's head.

'Hey boys!' I called out, 'I think you're missing something.'

'What?' asked Matthew.

I ushered Scott over to my bed, and, in a hushed voice, I told him, 'In my top drawer there are some glow-in-the-dark stickers of stars that one of my friends gave me. Take them.'

'Are you sure?' he asked.

'Absolutely.'

He smiled at me, opened the drawer, located the stickers and went back over to Matthew.

'Hey,' he said to Matthew, 'Kirsty reckons we should add

some of these to the space station.' He showed him the sheet of stars.

'Awesome!' Matthew exclaimed.

Scott stood on a chair and began sticking them on the ceiling above Matthew's bed. I don't think he should have been sticking them directly on the ceiling, but he didn't seem worried about getting into trouble. Maybe Scott was actually an angel inside the body of a human. He stuck down the last star and hopped down from the chair.

'This is the best space station ever!' Matthew's justifiably bad mood had floated away.

About an hour later, Mum and Matthew's mum returned and they both stared, puzzled, at all the plastic cups that were on the floor. Mum looked at me and I just shrugged. Then they both noticed the space station above Matthew's bed.

'Wow,' said Mum, 'that's pretty incredible.'

'I know,' said Matthew, beaming. 'Scott made it for me and Kirsty gave me glow-in-the-dark stars. You can already see them shining. They'll look so good at midnight.'

* * *

At midnight, Scott came to check on me and Matthew. I was wide awake, listening to Matchbox 20 on the Discman Dad had brought me.

'How are you doing, Kirsty?' he asked quietly.

'I'm okay. The central line is just sore. Listen, I just wanted to tell you that I think what you did for Matthew today was really cool.'

He smiled a strange smile at me.

'What?' I asked him.

'I was about to say the same thing to you.'

CHAPTER 26

Snugglepot and Cuddlepie

'Time to drop your daks,' said Danielle.

After several weeks of chemotherapy, I was home. I'd need to have more chemo, but we had to find a bone marrow match first. Danielle, Brett and Matthew had all had blood tests to see if they would be a match. They had tested Mum and Dad as well, even though it was unlikely either of them would be a match. I think the chances of a parent being a match for their child is about one in two hundred, because a child inherits half their genes from each parent. The chance of there being a match for me on the Bone Marrow Registry from a total stranger who was unrelated to me was one in a million. Dr Sue had sent me home, on a cloud of morphine, to wait for the results. A dream-like fuzz cradled my body and sketched a goofy grin on my face. Alongside this opiate euphoria was an itchy sensation on my skin.

'Great,' I said, my words dribbling with sarcasm, 'you'll get to see me naked.' I let out a swollen exasperated sigh.

Danielle ignored me and shut the bathroom door.

The bathroom had hard brown carpet covering every inch of the floor, which Dad had glued himself. He said carpet was safer as us kids might slip on wet tiles. The wallpaper had been chosen by Mum, and Mum and Dad had hung it together. It was a cream colour sprinkled with images of Snugglepot and Cuddlepie and lots of green gumtree leaves. The gumnut babies seemed rather happy to live on the walls of our bathroom.

As I squished my bottom onto the cold plastic toilet seat, goose bumps exploded all over my arms and legs. Each goose bump felt like an ant bite on my skin. Danielle turned on the bathtub taps and water roared out of them. 'Arms up,' she instructed me. Carefully, she pulled my t-shirt off.

I hugged my arms around my chest and concealed my tiny A-cup boobs from my bossy big sister. Her hands gripped my shoulders as she helped me to stand and shuffled me to the edge of the bathtub. The taps blasted more and more water into the brown bathtub and the bathroom began to steam up. Some of my goose bumps ceased chomping on my skin.

Whoosh!

My grey trackpants and my knickers had been ripped down from my hip bones to my ankles. 'Oh my god, Kirst ...' Danielle stepped away from me like she'd just spotted a python in the bathroom and not her little sister. Her eyes grew wide as she swallowed in my nakedness. 'You've got so skinny.'

She helped me into the hot soothing water. The goose bumps dissolved as I sat in the tub. I soaked up the euphoric buzz of opiates in my bloodstream.

'You kind of look like Kate Moss,' said Danielle. 'You know how she has that really skinny, waif-like body.'

'I wish I looked like Kate Moss.'

Danielle grabbed a blue sponge and began plunging it into the hot water, then picking it up and squeezing it so hot water gushed down my back, all while being careful not to let the water trickle down my chest and onto my central line. Oh, what stunning, steamy, welcome warmth after the hospital bird baths.

The bathwater had grown deeper. As it crept its way up my lower back and hips, the pain started. Needle holes in my back from attempted lumbar punctures stung as the hot water met with them. My right hip, which had been punched with countless biopsy needles, began to thump and pulse.

'Do you want me to wash your hair?' she asked.

'Yes!' I replied. 'It's filthy and it's not going to fall out yet. I can tell by the way it feels.'

Using a green jug from the kitchen, Danielle started pouring that heavenly hot water over my hair. She squeezed apple-scented shampoo on top of my head and began massaging the cold goo into my hair and my scalp. I wasn't cold any more. All my goose bumps had disappeared.

'I totally think I'm going to be a bone marrow match for you,' she said.

'I hope someone is.'

'What happens if no one is a match?'

A damp silence fell over our bathroom. Danielle rinsed the shampoo from my hair with the jug. She squeezed a generous dollop of conditioner into her hands, smooshed it into my scalp and began to comb it through my soon-to-be-gone long blonde hair. The comb soothingly scraped my back as it glided through my hair. Then she rinsed out the conditioner.

'Dr Sue said they'll need to give me at least three years of chemotherapy if I can't have a bone marrow transplant,' I said.

'Three years?!'

'Yeah ... and there's only about a seventeen per cent chance the chemotherapy will even work, so if I don't have a match for a bone marrow transplant then ...' I didn't need to finish the sentence.

People are expecting me to die this time.

'I'll give you a few minutes on your own.' She stood up and turned off the taps. Water stopped gushing into the tub, but my lower back and my hips still had a creature of pain wrapped tightly around them. She shut the door behind her.

I was alone with Snugglepot and Cuddlepie, the steamy bathwater and my morphine haze.

Then something caught my eye …

What the …?

There were little orange leaves floating on the surface of the bathwater near my feet. Then I realised there was something far stranger than leaves in the bathroom. I stared.

Is there a small girl with wings sitting on the edge of the bathtub with her feet swinging back and forth in the water?

The tiny girl's wings looked like they'd been plucked off a giant butterfly, and there were a few pink and white flowers in her long tangled blonde hair. She looked up at me and smiled. I shut my eyes.

Oh dear … this can't be a good sign. This isn't happening. I'm going to open my eyes on the count of three and it's just going to be me alone in the bathtub. One, two, three!

I opened my eyes.

She was still there, swinging her legs back and forth and humming to herself. I could *see* her and I could *hear* her. She pointed at the leaves near her feet. I lifted my arm up and pointed at them too. She chuckled softly.

Is she giggling at me?

'Knock, knock. Kirst, it's just me.'

I looked at Danielle as she opened the door, waiting to see her reaction to the fairy sitting on the edge of our bathtub.

'Are you ready to get out?'

I turned to look at my new winged friend.

She's gone!

'Did you hear me? I said, are you ready to get out?' Danielle asked again, as she unfolded a yellow towel and held it wide open and ready to throw around me.

'Yep,' I replied.

I stood up and, as Danielle swaddled me in the lavender-smelling towel, I realised the invisible pain entity was no longer wrapped around my body any more.

'Kirst? Are you feeling all right?'

'Um ...' I decided to lie. 'I was just remembering that when my hair falls out I'll lose my eyebrows and eyelashes as well ...'

'Really?' asked Danielle. '*All* of your hair falls out? Like, hair from *everywhere*?'

'Yep, all of it,' I said.

'What's that in the bathwater?' Danielle pointed near where the fairy had been sitting.

I looked. The water in the bath was now soapy and white and frothy, but there was definitely some flaky orange stuff floating on the surface.

Oh my gosh! The fairy left her leaves behind! She was real! I can tell Danielle all about her because she left proof that she was here.

Danielle stepped closer to the bathtub. 'Hey,' she said, 'this kind of looks like ...' She reached her hand down towards the water — then she suddenly jerked it backwards. 'Oh my god, Kirst ... Are these your *pubes*?'

'*What?!*' I shrieked. I looked down at my crotch and, sure enough, just beneath my white tummy was where my pubic hair *used* to be. The hair on my head and my eyebrows and eyelashes were all still attached, but my pubic hair had disappeared. 'You almost touched my floating pubes!' I teased her.

'Shut up! I didn't know what it was!'

We laughed together as she helped me step out of the tub.

'Pull the plug out for me, will you?' I told her.

'No way! I'm not putting my hand in there with your pubes!'

I leaned down and ripped the plug out. The gurgling was loud and abrupt and we laughed even more as we watched clumps of my wiry fire-coloured pubes get slurped down the plug hole. The drain made an especially loud noise at one point.

'Oh no,' she said, 'the plughole is choking on your pubes.'

CHAPTER 27

Sticky Air

'Are you sure you're up to this?'

'Yeah, Mum. I'll be right.'

'It's about thirty-three degrees today. Maybe you should wait until tomorrow — it might be cooler.'

'Nah, I'm ready to do this now.'

'All right, love.'

I'd been home for a few days and it was official — I was a bald cancer patient ... again. I had been told, once again, not to make my education a priority, and again I had decided to keep going to school as often as I could and arrange to get work from my teachers so I could keep up with my peers. Having missed several weeks of term, I was eager to go back to school again and see my friends. But first, I needed to familiarise everybody with this altered version of myself. They'd all been warned I'd be bald and very sick, but warnings and reality aren't ever the same. I knew I had to show them. I had to acclimatise my fellow teenagers as quickly as possible so we could move on.

It was a scorching hot day in February and my plan was to visit during lunchtime before I returned to attend classes. Like ripping off a Band-Aid — best done swiftly — I was going to show them what cancer-Kirsty looked like. No one, not even Debbie, had seen the reality of a chemo-cursed body up close before. I would give them a close-up. Let them stare. Let them take it all in. Let them be shocked, scared or disgusted, or all three.

I was wearing my favourite 'Sun, surf and smiles' t-shirt. It covered my central line, but it didn't cover my baldness, and nothing could conceal my puffy, pimply, steroid-inflamed cheeks. I had no eyebrows and no eyelashes. Every inch of my body was completely hairless — as Danielle could confirm. As I got out of the cool comfort of Mum's air-conditioned Camry, the heat sent ripples of sweat across my skin. The bell would ring for lunchtime soon — I'd timed it that way.

'Get someone to call me when you want me to come back and get you,' instructed Mum. 'Don't you dare try to make your own way home in this heat.'

I rolled my eyes. 'Yes, Mum.' I shut the door. She drove off. I was alone. It was a somewhat odd feeling. I didn't really get to be alone for longer than a few minutes at a time these days.

The sun blasted down on me as I stepped through the school gate. Nobody was around. They were all in class. Aside from arriving at lunchtime, I didn't really have a plan.

Maybe I should just sit and wait around the bench seats where my friends always hang out …

'Kirsty? Kirsty, is that you?' It was a guy in my grade called Ahmed. He approached me timidly.

'Hey, Ahmed,' I said.

'What are you doing here?'

'Oh, I just wanted to drop in and say "hello" to everyone.'

'Cool … um … I was just heading to the dunnies to have a smoke, but do you want me to go and get Debbie? We're in maths at the moment.'

'Yeah, that would be great. Sorry to interrupt your smoke break.'

He laughed nervously. 'That's okay.' But he didn't move. He just stood there, frozen, for a few moments. I let him be a statue while his brain clicked and turned and processed the horror of cancer. The sun was relentless. If I got burned, Mum would chuck a mental.

After a few awkward seconds, I said, 'Listen, it's really hot so I'm going to head up to the gym. Can you let Debbie and everyone know that I'm here and that I'd like to see them?'

'Sure. Of course.' He unfroze. 'It's great to see you,' he added, a clear sign of the good manners his parents had instilled in him. Off he went to get my friends and anyone else who might like the opportunity to see what a dying teenager looked like.

I slowly sauntered the few metres to the gym. The heat was less brutal indoors. The gym smelt like dirty socks and chalk. A big pile of navy mats were stacked up against the wall on my right. On my left were rows of chairs. I grabbed one and placed it in the centre of the room facing the doorway and sat down. Sweat puddles grew in my armpits. My heartbeat was steady. I sucked in a big deep breath through my nose and let it out of my mouth. It echoed in the empty space.

BRRRRRRRRRRRIIIIIINNNNNNNNNNNNNNNN NNNNNGGGGGGGGGGGG!!!

The bell for lunch rang. I had missed that sound. Suddenly, I heard clumsy footsteps. Someone was coming.

'Holy shit, Kirst …' It was Jane.

'Hey,' I said casually.

'Oh my god! I can't believe you're here.' As she came towards me, her eyes grew large and sad. I stood up. 'How are you feeling?'

'Umm …'

'Probably like shit. Probably like you have cancer or something.'

I laughed and found myself hugging her. I'd never hugged Jane before and I don't know why I did then. Maybe I was relieved that she was still being her usual funny self; that even though I looked so different, Jane wouldn't be treating me any differently. I felt her hugging me back.

'The others will all be here any minute,' she said.

Geoff and Ashley came in. I hugged both of them. Debbie came. I hugged her too. My body seemed to be instigating these hugs and I just let it happen.

Then, to my shock, in came the mean girls who'd bullied me in Year 8. My body even insisted on hugging them as well. Debbie and Jane stood on either side of me like two protective gargoyles as the gym began to fill with every student in our whole grade. My body made no exceptions — it hugged everyone that came through that door. I even hugged Mrs Ivers, the food technology teacher, and Mrs Griffiths, the drama teacher.

'Does your mother know you're here?' asked Mrs Ivers. 'She must be worried sick.'

'Yeah, she knows. She dropped me off,' I reassured her. 'She told me to call when I'm ready to be picked up.'

She pulled a classic 'I'm not impressed' teacher face. 'Hmm ... you should be at home resting.'

I turned to Debbie. 'Does Jake know I'm here?'

'Yeah,' answered Jane, 'I think everyone knows you're here. I'm sure he'll be here soon.'

I had to sit back down. I hadn't been among a crowd of people like this since our Year 10 formal.

'I'm going to go and get you a glass of water,' said Mrs Ivers. As she left, in dawdled Jake. He searched the gym with his eyes.

He doesn't recognise me. He's looking for the familiar Kirsty, but I'm not her any more.

Then shock splintered across his face.

I've seen this look before. It's the same look Amos had when he saw me as a bald little cancer girl. Now, here I am, a teenage cancer girl being stared at with the same expression of terror and despair.

It took him a long time to approach me. I stood up and hugged him, just as I'd hugged everyone else, but he didn't hug me back. Now I knew what the phrase 'stunned mullet' meant.

Mrs Ivers returned with my glass of water. Nausea wriggled in my belly. I sipped the water and tried to listen to Jane complain about how much homework there was in Year 11. Jake wasn't saying anything. He was standing about two metres away from me, still giving me that same look. His arms seemed as though they were made of overcooked spaghetti.

I knew then that things were over with Jake. Sometimes a look can say a thousand words, but his look simply said one word to me: 'no'.

And it wasn't just Jake. The gym was so filled with fear, it was as if it had solidified the air. When I gently moved my fingers, the air felt sticky, as though I'd stuck my hand inside a bag of fairyfloss.

It's a strange thing to be in a room where everyone is thinking the same thing about you. I felt their thoughts through the stickiness they'd created with their fear: *She's going to die. Kids that get cancer twice usually die.*

They had all accepted my hugs because they thought they were hugs goodbye. I wanted to show them they were all wrong.

CHAPTER 28

Sisters

I am a mistress of the art of vomiting. Vomit and I go a long way back. We have an understanding that while vomiting is indeed a necessary facet of my life, I will not cease to do the things that I want to do just because a vomit demands to make an appearance. It's a shame there's no prize for being an expert *vomiteur* because from a very young age I could successfully attend all my classes *and* still make time to spew several times a day.

On one such day in Year 11, I was sitting in English class with Mr Small when suddenly a vomit gave me a polite warning that it was on its way. I raised my hand.

'Yes?' said Mr Small, with a tone noticeably softer than the one he used for the rest of the class.

'May I please go to the bathroom?' I asked.

'Yes. Do you need to take someone with you?' he asked with concern slopped all over his face.

A few of my friends sat up straight, hoping I would say "yes" so they could get out of English for a few minutes, but I don't allow audiences to watch me vomit. It's a solitary activity.

'No. It's okay,' I reassured him, as I pushed my chair back, and my friends sank down into their seats. Mr Small still had some worry dribbling down his chin, but I had already begun to make my way towards the door. A crucial part of a successful vomit is the timing. You must allow adequate time to get your head safely positioned over the toilet bowl.

The toilet block was an ugly cement building down the bottom of the school near the basketball courts. It had rusty metal gates that were chained and locked up outside of school hours. As I got closer to this concrete monstrosity, the smell of urine and cigarette smoke whacked me across the face and my vomit threatened to come out prematurely. It didn't. I'm a professional.

I leaned on a cool metal railing for a few seconds, then, relying on experience and determination, strode down the stairs that led into the toilets. I clutched my stomach with contorted fingers as I walked past the sinks. Most of the taps were broken and there was never any soap to wash your hands. Almost all the toilet doors had broken locks. I'd figured out from previous vomit sessions which toilet doors had working locks and which ones hadn't. Unfortunately for me, the only doors that seemed to lock properly were right near the end of the block.

I bashed the blue graffitied door open with my shoulder, slammed and locked it behind me, and fell to my knees. The floor was sticky with years of urine. As my kneecaps knocked onto the floor, a jarring *bang* vibrated through my body, rattling my skeleton. Blue and purple imprints began to stain my knees. My tummy shook with spasms. My insides felt like tangled Christmas lights. My head throbbed, and sweat oozed out of my bald head.

I had barely positioned my face over the toilet when out into the world came a hideous, slimy, metallic mix of vomit, snot and tears. As my spew aggressively hit the water in the toilet bowl, the water retaliated and leapt at my face. I had filthy school dunny water on my face, but I didn't recoil. Clear snot flowed out of my nostrils. A handful of tears made salty tracks down my cheeks. The tracks ended near my chin and then joined the mixture of vomit, toilet water and snot.

At first, my vomit had been a mouth-twisting recipe of the water and tablets I'd had earlier that day. Then I began throwing up the bright-orange bitter gunk that I always seemed to throw up when my belly was empty. Big dollops of blood started dropping into the toilet. A nosebleed had joined my vomit party.

Whoever designed the human body certainly put *a lot* of holes in our face. Every orifice on my face was expelling something. More vomit, more tears and more drips of blood. I kept my head down and let the necessary unfold. My head felt like a brick and my delicate neck screamed as it struggled to hold up my enormous fluid-spewing skull. I could no longer smell cigarettes or urine. The pea-sized crimson drops falling from my nose became a steady stream of deep dark-red liquid. The cold from the floor was piercing into my knees. Between gagging up gunk, which had now turned yellow, I tried to take in gasps of air, but it was hard to breathe with both my mouth and nose otherwise occupied.

A few more seconds of time slipped away and I graduated from vomiting to dry-retching. My guts were empty, but my brain hadn't got the message yet. It would soon. My heart was running erratically. My head felt like someone had built a bonfire on top of my bulbous baldness. I could feel prickles of sweat erupting all over my back, making my school shirt damp and sending icy darts up and down my arms and legs. The gags slowed. The scarlet stream from my nose transformed into a dribble and then a few final plip-plops.

I reached over to my right and pulled out a massive long strip of the thinnest and cheapest toilet paper in the world. The worst part was over. The vomit had had its way and now it was time to put myself back together.

'Are you all right in there, sister?'

I fell backwards onto my bum in exhaustion and looked up at a face that was peering down at me over the wall of the toilet cubicle.

'Ah, sister, you don't look so good.' Another voice spoke and another head popped into sight, staring down at me.

'Should we go and get someone for you, sister?' Then, there was another.

'She doesn't look good.' A fourth fretful face shone its concern down onto me.

It was a quartet of Kirinari girls. Kirinari was the Aboriginal hostel that was near our school.

'I'm all right,' I said, as I wiped my face with a scrunched handful of toilet paper. 'I just need to sit here for a minute.'

'Open the door and we'll sit with you,' said one of the girls.

'You don't need to do that. You should go back to class,' I said.

'Nah, open up and we'll sit with you.'

One of them began knocking on the door, calling out, 'Knock, knock, who's there?' They all giggled.

I examined the graffiti on the back of the door. There were three statements that were legible: 'LL is a dud root,' 'RC has a small dick' and 'NJ is a slut guts'. Each time I came here to vomit, I hoped that someone would have written a new comment for me. I blew my nose and wiped my eyes and face with another handful of transparent, rough-textured toilet paper. I reached up, unlocked and swung open the toilet door. We all sat on the floor together.

'You're that chick in Tyson's year, aren't you?' asked one of my new friends.

'Ah, you just wanna talk about Tyson 'cause you're in love with him!' teased one of the girls.

'Nah, she is!'

'Yeah, she's the chick with cancer. That's you, isn't it?'

'Yep, that's me.'

'We'll help ya get up off the floor.' The Tyson–lover extended her hand towards me, gripped my small wrist and lifted me to my feet. They escorted me to the sinks. I made a cup with my hands and washed my face with soothing cool water. I made another cup and slurped the liquid into my mouth, rinsing out any remnants of chunder that tried to stay behind.

'We'll walk you back to class, sister.'

My new friends walked with me and talked, cracking up laughing every few seconds. I felt like a balloon after someone has blown it up, then let go of it, and left it deflated on the floor, a squishy mess covered in someone's spit that no one in their right mind would want to pick up. Yet I found myself cackling along with the girls. Laughter is far more pleasant than chuck when it roars out of your mouth. I unzipped the pocket in my school skirt and took out a packet of chewing gum. I unwrapped a piece and popped it into my mouth, moving it around my teeth and all over my tongue to destroy the bitterness and ick-factor that vomiting had left there. I offered gum to the girls and they each took a piece. We paused for a minute near my classroom, chewing our gum.

'Thanks for walking with me,' I said.

'Ya don't need to thank us, sister.'

'Hey, why do you keep calling me "sister"?' I asked them.

'It's because you *are* our sister,' said the tallest girl, like I was a total airhead who'd just asked a silly question.

'What do you mean?' I asked.

'You're Koori, sister!'

'Koori?' I still didn't get it.

'Yeah, Koori? Aboriginal.'

'I am?'

They all cackled.

'Didn't you know?'

'But ... how could you know that about me?'

She gave me a knowing smile. 'Have you ever tried asking your mum?'

'She doesn't really talk about her ancestors and we don't really see her family.'

They all thought this was hysterical.

'Then you're definitely one of us, sister. Ask your mum. She'll probably get the shits. She may never admit it and you may not have known it, but you're a sister, sister.'

Exhausted from my trip to the toilets, I stood for a moment in the hallway outside of my classroom.

'We'll see ya 'round, sister,' said the Tyson-lover, and with that they took off down the corridor.

Is this why Mum never wants to see her family? Because they're Aboriginal? What's wrong with being Aboriginal? Why would she hide it from me or Danielle, Brett and Matthew?

* * *

When I arrived home from school, Mum was leaving to take Brett to soccer training. As soon as I heard the car pull out of the driveway, I went and got her address book. I found a phone number for Uncle Les. My heart began pounding as I dialled the number.

A man answered.

'Hi, this is Kirsty. Jill's daughter. I wanted to speak to Uncle Les.'

'Kirsty!' The man's voice filled with joy. 'It's me! It's so good to hear from you. We heard you're sick again, but I haven't been able to get hold of your mum so we can come and visit you. How are you? Are you okay?' His voice suddenly sounded panicked. He must've thought I was calling with bad news about my cancer.

'I'm doing okay. Listen, I wanted to ask you something. There were some girls at school today ... some Aboriginal girls. They told me that I'm Aboriginal.'

Silence.

'Are you still there?' I asked.

'Yeah, darlin', I'm still here.'

'Is it true? Am I Aboriginal?'

More silence. Then, 'Have you spoken to your mum about this?'

'No. I wanted to speak to you first.'

A longer silence lurched along.

'Yes,' he said eventually, 'your grandmother, my mum and your mum's mum, was Aboriginal, and that means you are

Very faintly, I could hear magpies singing in our backyard.

'Well, at school today some girls from Kirinari told me I'm Aboriginal and I called Uncle Les and he said it's true.'

'When did you call Uncle Les?'

'About ten minutes ago.'

'Well, your uncle smokes marijuana so I think he gets things confused sometimes. Look at Danielle and Brett. They've got orange hair and fair skin with freckles. Your hair, when you had it, was the fairest out of all you kids. And you've got the whitest skin as well.'

'Matthew has dark hair and dark skin and dark eyes,' I stated.

'So?' She was getting testy.

'Well ... why does Matt have darker colouring than the rest of us?' I asked. 'Your colouring is dark like Matthew's as well.'

'It's because there's Italian blood on my side of the family.' Mum was officially pissed off and the conversation was over. We stared at each other.

I think she's lying.

The magpies continued their uproar outside.

Why would she lie to me?

CHAPTER 29

The Good, the Bad and the Ugly

One of the many things that I adored about the Sutherland Shire was that I could walk anywhere I wanted or needed to be and I always had the gumtrees to keep me company. But there came a day when my tree friends abandoned me.

Going to school in Year 11 and 12 while being on chemotherapy was difficult, but I don't think people knew the full extent of my difficulties as I always put on a brave front. I went to as many classes as I could. I painted confidence on my face for my teachers, even the ones that gave me pity-soaked 'you're going to die' smiles. I was sure to reassure anyone who made eye contact with me that I was going to be okay.

Debbie, Jane, Geoff and Ben were the best friends that anyone could ask for. Their loyalty to me never faltered. I also had my newfound 'sisters', the Kirinari girls — I didn't even mind vomiting at school any more because they were usually loitering in the dunnies and would keep me company. But, as I had learned back in primary school, there are always nasty bullies, and having cancer didn't dissuade them from being cruel to me. I tried to ignore the mean comments people made, sometimes within earshot, and sometimes behind my back.

'Oh my god! She looks like a total freak. Why doesn't she wear a wig or something so we don't have to look at her? It's depressing for us to have to see that.'

'What's she even coming to school for? My mum said that when someone gets cancer twice, they always end up dying. Why bother with school if you're just going to die?'

'Look how white she is. She looks so gross.'

Then, as if the comments weren't cutting enough, they'd laugh at me too. It seemed my cancer and bald head were amusing to some.

I would make it through to last period and, as the bell shrieked, I'd start to feel a sense of accomplishment, relieved that all I needed to do now was walk the short distance home. I would make my way down Hotham Road and the ghost gums would protect me and they wouldn't comment on my cancer and they would certainly never laugh at my bald head.

On one particularly exhausting day, my feet felt prickly and numb from chemo, so I was especially eager to head home after the last-period bell. With my tingling feet, I began striding away from school.

'Kirst! Wait up!' It was Jake.

I was surprised. He had been avoiding me as if cancer was contagious. Reluctantly, I waited outside the metal gates.

He jogged towards me. 'Hey, I just wanted to ask you something. I'll walk home with you.'

'Okay,' I replied. I set off homewards, with Jake sauntering along beside me.

Something's wrong.

'I wanted to ask you what mark you got for our *Macbeth* essay in English,' he said.

I couldn't hear the gum leaves breathing overhead. *Why are they silent today? They're hardly ever silent.* My mouth tasted like my lunch — mercaptopurine tablets and the gagging tin flavour of Panadeine Forte.

'I got eighteen out of twenty,' I said.

'Seriously?'

'Yeah, why? What did you get?'

He didn't answer. 'Are you coming to school tomorrow?' he asked.

'No. I've got to have a lumbar puncture tomorrow and some other treatment. It will take all day, so I won't make it to school.'

'Oh ...'

'So what mark did you get?'

Again, he ignored the question. We walked a few more steps under the silent gumtrees.

'Come on,' I said, 'I told you my mark.'

'Seven out of twenty,' he confessed. 'How did you get eighteen? I tried really hard and stayed up late working on it, but I totally stuffed it up. Do you think I could take a look at your essay? Or maybe you could explain to me how you got such a high mark?'

'Um … yeah. Maybe. This is weird,' I blurted out.

'What's weird?'

'You know. You barely talk to me or look at me and now you want me to help you because you don't know how to write an essay on your own.'

Surprise rippled across his face. 'Kirst … What's wrong?'

'Why don't you just admit it? You hate being near me. You hate the sight of me now that I'm sick.'

I stopped walking and plonked down, butt first, onto the footpath. My left bum cheek was on the grass and I could feel sharp bindies stabbing into the back of my thigh. My right bum cheek was on the hot scratchy surface of the leafless footpath. Jake plonked down on my right. My eyes stared down deeper and deeper below the footpath and into the dirt of the earth. Jake was looking down too.

'Last year, you chased me home and kissed me,' I said. 'Then I got cancer. I warned you so many times that it would be bad and you kept saying you wanted to stick by me and be my boyfriend, but as soon as you saw me with my bald head …

you barely come near me. I know you don't like me any more because I've got cancer. I'm right, aren't I?'

'Yes!' he yelled. He put his hands over his ears.

'Are you scared I'm going to die?'

'No.'

'Is it because of how I look?'

'Yes! Yes, it's because of how you look! I know you warned me, but I had no idea that you would look so … so … *so ugly!* You don't even look like you! I'm trying to be a good person, but I just can't stand the way you look. You look so bad, Kirst. Kids at school are saying you look like a freak. I know this means I'm a bad person, but I can't help the way I feel. I hate looking at you now that you're like this. I can't stand seeing the back of your head when you're walking down the corridors to class. And your face! What's happened to your face?! You look so different.'

I didn't know what to say. We sat there on the ground. The ghost gums weren't helping me. No one was helping me. Bindies pierced my left hand as I pushed myself up and onto my feet. I reached out my right hand to help Jake to his feet. He didn't take it.

'Come on,' I said. 'You need to get home or you'll get in trouble and I need to get home or Mum is going to start to worry about me.' I hooked my thumbs under the straps of my backpack.

He dragged his body up from the ground and, suddenly, his face fumed with fury. 'I'm really sick of you walking around like you're better than everyone else. You need to think about the way you're acting and what people are thinking about you. You need to stop pretending that you don't have cancer.' Rage spread over his face and, for a few moments, Jake didn't look like himself at all. He'd morphed into a mutilated troll.

'What do you mean I walk around like I'm better than everyone else?'

'You know what I mean. The way you always have to come to school all the time, even when you're so sick. Why do you do that?' he ranted at me, his face inches from mine. 'I don't know what you're trying to prove!'

'You don't know what I'm trying to prove?' I said incredulously, my own anger awakening. 'I'm not trying to prove anything! I'm trying to finish high school and do my HSC and not die from cancer at the same time. Do you have any idea how hard this is for me?' Tears crept into my voice. 'I need to go home.'

I left Jake on the footpath. As I trudged home, I didn't hear a single leaf rustle. I looked up to check the trees were still there. They were there, but they were totally quiet.

Before I even reached for the doorknob, Mum swung the front door open. She'd been waiting for me to get home from school.

'What's wrong, love? Are you in pain? I need to talk to you about something.'

'I was talking with Jake after school.' I pushed past her and headed towards my bedroom. Mum followed me.

'What's wrong? I can tell something's wrong.'

Please leave me alone, Mum. I just want to go in my room and do my Ancient History homework.

I made it to my doorway, Mum still by my side. I dropped my backpack down near my desk.

'Kirsty, love, tell me ...'

I couldn't hold it in. There was an electrical storm inside me and I couldn't contain it. 'Jake told me the reason he doesn't like me any more is because cancer has made me look ugly.'

'What? Did he actually say that?'

'Yep, he said he doesn't think about me dying, he just has a problem with how I look.' I slid down onto my bedroom floor. I held on to my ugly cancer head with both hands and pulled my knees into my chest.

'Oh, love ...' Mum put her arm around my shoulders for a few seconds, but she wasn't much of a hugger; that was Dad's field of expertise. 'I got a couple of phone calls today. Matthew from hospital died and Dr Sue wants you to call her. I'll go and get you a cold face washer. Don't cry.' Mum left me for a few minutes and came back with a wet yellow face washer. 'Here, love, wipe your face.'

I couldn't move. Mum began wiping the cool cloth over my bald head and around the back of my neck. I squeezed my eyes shut. Scalding tears oozed out of them. I couldn't hold them in any more. Mum wiped my flushed face. 'Here, blow your nose.' She shoved a handful of tissues towards me. I drenched the tissues in so much snot that Mum had to give me another handful. 'Come on, take a deep breath.' I could only breathe through my mouth. My nose was too blocked. 'I'm going to get you a nice cold drink of cordial.' Off Mum went and I sat there with my mountain of soiled tissues. Mum returned quickly with a big plastic cup of orange cordial in one hand and a medicine cup in the other. 'You've got to take your afternoon tablets, love.'

I began taking my afternoon snack of yellow and white tablets one at a time with my faithful orange cordial. Mum waited for me to finish and took the cup from me.

'Do you want anything to eat?'

'No thanks, Mum. I better call Dr Sue.'

* * *

'I'm so sorry, Kirsty,' said Dr Sue. 'None of your siblings are a match for you. There's no one on the registry who's a match either. We won't be able to give you a bone marrow transplant.' My ears started ringing. 'Unfortunately, our best chance of getting you into remission and keeping you there is three years of chemotherapy.' My body was standing in the hallway holding on to the phone, but my soul had slithered to the ground. It felt like it was melting and then evaporating into non-existence. 'The good thing is we can take out your central line and put in a portacath. Portacaths are sort of the same as central lines, but you can get them wet. You'll be able to have showers and go swimming.'

Three years of chemo. Matthew is dead. I'm an ugly cancer freak.

'I am very sorry about this, Kirsty. Kirsty? Are you still there?'

'Yeah, I'm still here.'

'We'll talk more in person when you come into hospital.'

'Okay. Bye.'

Mum had been standing in the hallway. I didn't need to tell her what Dr Sue had just told me — she knew.

'I've got homework to do,' I said.

'What? Love, don't worry about your homework today. Why don't you have a rest and watch some television? Someone is going to give us a call about Matthew's funeral. You don't have to go if you think it will be too much for you.'

'I'll be going,' I snapped. Of course I'd go.

'Okay, love. Are you sure you feel like doing your homework?'

'Yep, I have to. If I don't do my homework, then all I'll have to think about is how I'm an ugly cancer freak and that I've got *another* funeral to go to. I need to do my homework, Mum.'

She nodded.

'Mum? Do you remember when I was sick in primary school and those kids chased me and threw rocks and sticks at me and then that boy hit me in the head with his school bag?'

'Yes, love, I remember. I had to soak the blood out of your school uniform. Why?'

'I wish Jake had chased me and thrown rocks and sticks at me instead of saying what he said to me today.'

'Oh, love.' Mum gave me another one of her half-hugs. 'Danielle will be home soon and, once you do your homework, I think you should call Debbie. Debbie's been such a good friend to you.'

'Okay.'

I went to my bedroom, opened up my school bag and took out my Ancient History homework. I read about the Spartans and how strong they were. I read that the women were so tough they didn't make a sound during childbirth, and that they would cut off one of their breasts so they could be better at archery. I wished I was as strong as the Spartan women. I wished I had died instead of Matthew. I wished I didn't care that Jake thought I was ugly, but I did care and I still care. I still care about *everything*.

CHAPTER 30

We Are Going to Win

'I can't wait to get this thing out of me,' I said, lifting the two tubes that were part of my central line.

'And what are they putting inside you instead?' Debbie asked. She'd come over to visit me after my trifecta of terrible news.

'It's another intravenous tube inside my chest, which will be hooked up to a vein near my heart. But this tube won't hang on the outside of my body like this stupid thing, so I'll finally be able to have a proper shower and, more importantly, I'll be able to swim, and that means we can go ahead and win the Splash-a-thon this year.'

'How do they use it if it's underneath your skin?' she asked. 'Like, how do they get the chemo into you?'

'With a needle,' I said. 'Any time I have to have chemo, they'll pierce a needle through my skin in exactly the same spot.'

'So, you're going to feel the needle every time?' she asked, her face a collage of horror and disgust.

'Yeah,' I said. 'But it's okay. At least they'll get it right on the first go. I won't have to sit there and have some doctor try twelve times just to get a needle into a worn-out vein that's totally collapsed. The part of the tube that will get pierced with needles looks like a ball thingy ...'

'And you like balls?' Debbie grinned at her dirty joke.

'No!' I exclaimed. 'That is so gross! I was going to tell you that this round thingy is going to sit under the skin just below my left boob, so it will be like a mini third breast.' I giggled, imagining myself with three boobs.

'Seriously?'

'Yep, I'm going to have an extra boob.'

Debbie could make the worst day of your life seem like it wasn't so bad.

* * *

So ... the central line was removed from my body and replaced with a portacath. It hurt just as badly as the central line did when they'd put it in. After the surgery, I could not turn my head left or right, or look up or down. I could only look straight ahead.

'When can I go home?' I asked Mum.

'I think you have to stay overnight,' she said.

'I want to go home.'

'I know you do, love.'

I could feel where they'd sliced my skin open and put the new tube inside. It scorched and stung my flesh.

'Why don't we take you for a little walk around to the parents' room?' suggested Mum.

I swung my legs off the edge of the bed and stood up. Very slowly and in great agony, I shuffled to the parents' room, where I collapsed, sweaty and exhausted, onto the two-seater couch in the middle of the room.

'Do you feel like seeing a visitor?' Mum asked. 'She can't turn her head because of the surgery today,' Mum explained to the visitor standing in the doorway. My guest came and sat right next to me and grabbed hold of my left hand.

'Hi, Kirsty.' It was Wayne. Wayne wasn't exactly a close friend whom I'd see regularly. Our encounters had always been at fundraisers. The fact that he was sitting here with me at the hospital — well, I knew things must be bad. Really bad. Like I'm having three years of chemo kind of bad. Like everybody is terrified, but no one is talking about it kind of bad. Like people are thinking I'm going to die kind of bad.

Wayne sat there, silently holding my hand. Mum was jabbering away at him, saying it was nice of him to visit and how she knew what a busy man he was.

'Wayne,' I said quietly, 'my team is going to win the Splash-a-thon this year.'

He nodded, because what could he say? He wasn't going to admit that it was likely I would be dead soon. No one was going to say that — well, not to my face anyway.

'This year, my team is going to be called "The Water Faeries" and we're going to be the team that raises the most money,' I went on. 'We're even going to make more money than Laguna Street Public School.'

Wayne sat with me a little longer. Then, just before he left, he said something to Mum that surprised me. 'I know people always tell you, "If you need anything, just ask," but I want you to know that I actually mean it. If you or Kirsty or your family ever need anything, I want you to ask me, okay?'

'That's very nice of you, Wayne,' said Mum. 'Thank you. I'd better get Kirsty back to bed now.'

He squeezed my hand one last time. Mum ushered him out.

'I promise you, Wayne,' I said, as he disappeared from my view. 'My team are going to win this year.'

CHAPTER 31

Thunk!

At the age of eighteen, I was preparing for my final exams and I was getting ready for a funeral — just another regular day for me in the sunny Sutherland Shire. Today was the funeral of yet another young dead cancer comrade. The deaths wouldn't stop. I began to count them after Matthew's funeral. The one I was attending today — Luke's — was number eighteen.

I'd become very accustomed to attending funerals. Rituals like not wearing black, or releasing white doves or balloons or butterflies into the sky, had lost all significance — it was just what people did when the unfathomably wrong occurred. As many funerals as I had attended, I'd never been to the funeral of a person who had died of old age. Still, I thought I knew all there was to know about funerals, until ...

Thunk, thunk, thunk!

'You can touch him if you like.'

Thunk, thunk, thunk!

I wish she'd stop that.

'Can you hear that when I knock on him? He sounds hollow. Like a drum.'

Thunk, thunk, thunk!

Like she was knocking on someone's front door, Luke's mother rapped her knuckles against her dead son's torso. A plastic mannequin of a boy rested in front of me. As his mother tapped on his sternum, you could hear the emptiness inside the shell of the body. If you've ever knocked on the door of an empty house and heard the echo of bare floorboards answer you, then you can imagine the sound that still haunts me.

'Doesn't the embalming look good?'

No. This is horrifying.

'He looks like he's sitting in bed with his eyes shut.'

No, he doesn't. He looks like a corpse. That's a body with no soul left inside it.

'There's nothing to be afraid of.'

Yes, there is. I could be this corpse. I could be the next one. I could be number nineteen on the death scoreboard.

'Come in. Touch him. Talk to him. It's what he wanted.'

He wanted to live. Just like me. He was just like me.

Thunk, thunk, thunk!

I was a statue, frozen into stillness by what my eyes were consuming. For several enormous minutes, Mum and I stood in the doorway of his bedroom.

'I'll give you some time alone with him.'

I never want to be an embalmed corpse propped up in my bedroom with Mum knocking on my chest.

I finally moved, but only my eyes. I looked out the window and could see Luke's father and friends hammering nails into wood and spray-painting it with various colours. They were building a coffin in the driveway. I found myself wishing that they'd just decided to release some white doves instead.

'Goodbye, love,' Mum whispered to Luke and she went and kissed his embalmed forehead. 'I'm just going to wait outside the door,' she said quietly to me. 'Take as long as you want. I'll be right here.'

I mustered up my courage and walked slowly to the side of his bed. I whispered some words that were only for him.

'I'm sorry I'm alive and you're not. I don't know who decides who dies and who gets to live. Goodbye, Luke.'

I didn't touch him. I couldn't. I should've hugged him when he was alive. I should've spoken to him more when we were in hospital together, but now there was nothing I could do.

Sometimes, I still hear the *thunk* noise and wonder, *Why am I still here? All of those kids deserved to be alive, but they're not.*

CHAPTER 32

Water Faeries

I leaned against the rough bark of a tree outside the Sutherland Leisure Centre. The gentle whooshing and scraping sounds of the gumtrees, and my little brother, Matt, kept me company as I waited for Mum, Dad, Danielle and my friends.

Yesterday, it had taken the registrar fifteen attempts to get my lumbar puncture right, and then I'd had to have vincristine injected into my portacath. I could feel the vincristine smashing my body right now. It was just the same as when I'd had it as a kid. As soon as it was injected into me the poison made itself at home inside my veins, spreading. Its lethal taste swamped my mouth. It was the drug responsible for my hands and feet becoming riddled with pins and needles. It sent vindictive, jarring, crippling muscular spasms through my limbs. Without warning, it hurled electric bolts into my heart that then ricocheted under my skin. It slung jagged, catapulting pricks of pain deep into my core, but I denied its ability to disable me. I refused to be weak. I refused to show how much pain I was in to anybody.

Dr Sue had wanted me to stay in hospital yesterday. 'Just a day or two,' she'd said, but it was never a day or two once they had you in their clutches, so I told her I had plans for the weekend and wouldn't be able to stay.

'What are you doing this weekend?' she asked.

'My friends and family have raised thousands of dollars for the Children's Cancer Institute of Australia and we're swimming in a nine-hour Splash-a-thon tomorrow. We're a team. I have to be there.'

'How did you raise all of that money?'

'My whole team did, but it was mostly me and my best friend, Debbie. We went into every shop in the Sutherland Shire, told people what we were doing and they all gave us money. I think my bald head helped get money out of people.'

'I'm going to give you Panadeine Forte to help with the vincristine pain.'

I briskly walked out of there with Mum trailing behind me.

'Slow down, Kirsty!' Mum yelled at me, her voice echoing in the lengthy corridor that led to liberation — well, to the car park. 'We'll be driving in peak-hour traffic, so walking fast isn't going to get us home any faster!'

Mum was right, but I continued my victory charge towards the lifts anyway.

The bark on the tree was monstrous underneath my hand. I much preferred the smoothness of ghost gumtrees.

Twang!

A vincristine missile hit my body. I soundlessly clung to the tree.

Danielle, Mum and Dad would soon be arriving. Brett had decided he was going to stay at home this time. My friends would also be here any minute, and I knew their company would coincide with an inexplicable decrease in the intensity of pain my body was feeling, just as it always did.

Matt was singing 'Wannabe' to himself as he kicked at twigs and walked in circles around the tree that was helping me stand up.

I chuckled through my cement wall of agony. 'Are you singing a Spice Girls song?'

'Yep.'

'You can go and play on the swings over there if you're bored.'

'I'm not bored and Mum told me I had to watch you. She says you push yourself too hard. She says you shouldn't keep pushing all the time and that you try to do too much, like go to school and stuff.'

'What else does Mum say about me?'

Matt stopped kicking the ground. 'Are you going to die from cancer this time?'

'Did someone tell you that I'm going to die?'

'*Everyone* talks about it. Mum says that *all* the kids from hospital that relapse *always* end up dying.'

'What did you say when Mum said that?'

'I asked Dad if you were going to die because Mum said all those other kids had died and he said, "Mum doesn't know everything."'

* * *

A plane rumbled overhead among wisps of clouds as I got ready to swim. I inhaled the bouquet of bleach, chlorine and Jane's hot chips, which she'd smothered in salt and vinegar. Thanks to Debbie's mum, we were all wearing homemade tutus and fairy wings made of metal coat hangers and stockings that had been dyed with colour and stretched over the hangers. Debbie had allocated each of us a colour. I was blue. Ben was green, and he was certainly a committed fairy. The night before the swim, he'd peroxided his dark hair and then dyed it bright green especially for today. He was wearing an emerald-green shirt with white flowers on it, and green glitter from his wings twinkled on his tanned arms and hands.

It was my turn to swim. I dropped my body under the water and thrust forwards with my palms together and my arms pointed straight. Noiselessness scooped me into its embrace under the water. My portacath ached underneath my navy Mambo bathing suit. No bikini for me this year.

My head surfaced and the racket above the water rumbled around me. I began swimming breaststroke. With every dip under the surface, the crowd was muzzled. I noticed the lane ropes weren't as bright as they had been last year. They'd been faded by the sun.

Vincristine electrocuted me, terrifying my torso as I swam. Yet I kept on swimming, up and down, up and down. Jane was waiting at the end of the lane in her black bathing suit. 'Kirst!' she yelled out. 'You've been in there for ages! Let me get in!'

I shook my head and kept on swimming. Jane stood with her hands on her hips for a while, but eventually yelled out, 'All right! I'll come back in a bit!'

I've got to keep swimming. If I stop moving, I might end up like Melissa and Matthew and all the other kids.

A pain spear was suddenly hurled through my spine. Tears came and I paused to tread water for a few moments, but then I continued to swim.

'Kirst! It's been over an hour! You should get out!' Debbie called out.

'I'm fine, Debs!' I lied.

Why is everybody trying to get me out of the water? Why can't I just swim forever?

* * *

Hours had passed on the giant clock that Wayne had put up to count down the time. I was now a white wrinkly cancer girl warped with agony. As I swam closer to the shallow end, there was Danielle holding up something for me to see. As I got closer, I recognised my dear and necessary friend — Panadeine Forte. I nodded at Danielle. I *had* to stop swimming.

I heaved my body up and out of the pool. Geoff splashed in and said, 'Geez, Kirst. What's with hogging all the swimming?'

I refuse to be weak. I refuse to let the pain stop me.

As soon as I was out of the water, an explosion of goose bumps bit their teeth into my skin. Jane threw a big blue towel around me that she had been warming for me in the sunshine.

'You need to take some drugs and eat something,' Jane commanded, as she walked with me to the grassy knoll where my family and friends were camping for the day. I gulped down two tablets with a can of Coke. The opiates gently carried me into a euphoric sense of bliss.

* * *

'Attention everyone!' Wayne's voice boomed. The nine hours had passed. 'Our two top teams are absolutely neck and neck in terms of the amount of money they've raised. We just need a few extra minutes to count, so we can be sure of this year's winner!'

We all stood in the foyer of Sutherland Leisure Centre, excited to hear the results. Debbie was squeezing my right hand and Ben was squeezing my left hand.

'I *really* want us to win,' said Debbie, 'but it doesn't matter if we don't. We still raised a lot of money.'

'Nah, we're gonna win!' said Ben. He let go of my hand, took out his wallet and pulled out the lone fifty-dollar note inside. He strode over to Wayne, handed it to him, came back and grabbed hold of my hand again.

'All right,' said Wayne. 'Ladies and gentlemen, we have a winner, but before I announce which team that is, I wanted to let you all know that this year we've raised over forty thousand dollars for the Children's Cancer Institute of Australia. This is the most amount of money we've ever raised at this event.'

There was a resounding cheer. Ben and Debbie squished my fingers even tighter.

Wayne resumed: 'Earlier this year I went to visit a young lady in hospital and she said to me, "Wayne, the Water Faeries are going to win the Splash-a-thon this year." And Kirsty, it looks like you're the kind of girl who, when she says she's gonna do something, she does it. The Water Faeries are this year's winners!'

Another burst of applause and victory whistles clanged all around me. Hot salty blobs tumbled down my face as Wayne beckoned me over to where he was standing. As he hugged me, I whispered, 'I told you we'd do it.'

He handed me a giant gold trophy. I carried it over to my team of faeries. Jane took it from me and held it high in the air. Ben picked me up, hugged me, put me back on the ground, kissed the top of my head and said, 'You're incredible, Kirst. I wish you could see yourself the way I see you.'

CHAPTER 33

Patti's Class

One of my favourite smells is the scent of old books. I love the combination of dust, age and yellowed paper. I love the feeling of anticipation when I pick up a book I've never read, and knowing that that book may have beguiled the minds of countless people before coming to strike a path through my own brain. I feel a charge of electricity surge through me as I run my fingers over the texture of books. How much will I love the story inside? Will this be another writer that I'll need to cradle in my heart? I have a passion for Paul Jennings, Henry Lawson, Robert Frost, John Marsden, Roald Dahl and William Shakespeare, but I can always make room for another author. If I could, I'd snort the scent of old books instead of eating food, and be content forever.

The University of Sydney campus had this intoxicating book smell waiting to waft into my nostrils around almost every corner.

Walking around the sandstone buildings was so soothing — they'd put their feet into the ground so long ago and I could just tell they didn't care that I had cancer. I was here to soak in all I could at a life-writing course with a writer called Patti Miller.

I was now in my last year of school. Everyone continued to wonder why I insisted on doing my final exams when it was likely that I wouldn't survive three years of chemo. I had met lots of patients at hospital who, no matter what age they were, had dropped out of school as soon as they were told it was okay to do so. I don't know why I didn't do the same. I wasn't trying to be strong or brave. It just didn't feel like it was the right thing to do. Maybe I was simply trying to prove people wrong. Or maybe Mum was right and I was pushing myself too much. Maybe I *would* die and completing my English homework every day would've been a waste of time.

So, just in case I didn't survive, I thought I should write some things down. I decided I would write some stories for my friends and my family so they could remember me after I became another dead cancer kid.

The castle-like buildings awed me as I dawdled past them looking for the one that my classes would be in. I found it. It was in a small cottage-like building. The room was small. Chairs and tables had been arranged into a circle. I placed my bag on the floor and sat at one of the tables. I got out a crisp new notepad and a black Artline felt-tip pen — my favourite kind of pen to write with.

If you combined the mischief of a pixie and the elegance of Princess Diana, then you'd get a fairly accurate image of the stunning, wise and totally cool chick that is Patti Miller. She had flame-coloured hair and the sun had left her with a festival of freckles upon her cheeks. She was one of those women who had such a perfectly crafted face that she could pull off a short funky hairstyle. I liked her immediately because she smiled with her mouth and her eyes at the same time.

My classmates were men and women who were all over the age of sixty. At hospital, I was always the oldest, so it was nice to be the youngest for a change. And perhaps I was not as out of place as I looked among this group — they were living the latter part of their lives and maybe I was as well.

Our first task was to write about a time when we felt uncomfortable. Chemotherapy immediately handed me plenty of times of discomfort to choose from. I flicked through these files in my memory cabinet and chose one. I was about to start writing when a clean-shaven gentleman sitting on my left cleared his throat quietly to get my attention.

'Excuse me, young lady,' he said, 'but are you sure you're in the right class? You know, this is a *life*-writing course.'

'Yes, I'm sure.' I smiled, but he didn't smile back.

I frantically began scribbling down my story. After about fifteen minutes, Patti got each of us to read what we had written out loud.

A grey-haired woman who looked exactly like a quintessential grandmother — down to her pastel-pink cardigan and matching small leather handbag — went first. I couldn't wait to hear what fascinating things this woman would have to share with us. I was sure her story would be flooded with the wisdom of a lifetime of experiences.

She read. I listened. I couldn't believe it. She told us the story of losing her virginity — in extremely graphic detail.

The gentleman who didn't return smiles went next. He told us a story about watching his friend die in the Vietnam War. As he read, I forgave him for not smiling back. The poor man had had all his smiles stolen from him.

My turn. I read my story about having a lumbar puncture. They were the most uncomfortable things I'd endured as a child and were still just as horrifying now as an eighteen-year-old. I finished reading and the room was silent.

Then Mr Stolen Smiles asked, 'Is that fiction you've just read?'

'No, it's real. It happened in the past and it's happening now.'

'Not bad,' he said, and he winked at me. He still didn't give away any smiles, but I now understood that he didn't have any to give and he now understood why I had to be here.

CHAPTER 34

He Loves Me. He Loves Me Not. He Loves Me?

My body was trying to tell me something. I could feel a relentless buzzing whirring around my bloodstream. My bones were screaming at me.

On top of that, Mum was letting Uncle Les come to visit. She never liked her brother to visit, so I could make an educated guess as to why he had received this rare invitation.

I'm close to dying.

I knew what everybody was saying when I wasn't around — 'She's not going to make it.' I glided along like I was already an apparition. I felt like I was in a strange realm between existence and death. Uncle Les coming to visit only confirmed what my body was preparing me for.

When he arrived at the house, I gave him a hug. His hair was the colour of midnight when there's no moon or stars, and his skin was the same hue as Matthew's. He was wearing a black t-shirt with the Aboriginal flag on it. Mum swiftly glanced in disapproval at his t-shirt, then went to make cups of tea for herself, Dad and Uncle Les. She put the cups and a packet of Iced Vovo biscuits on the dining-room table.

'How are you feeling, darling?' Uncle Les asked me, with a whiff of cigarettes emanating from his mouth.

I said what I usually said: 'I'm okay.'

'She's pushing herself too hard trying to get to school all the time, and a friend of hers from hospital died recently.' Mum's voice was pulled tight like a rubber band.

'Are you still doing your singing and drama classes?' asked Uncle Les. I was surprised to discover that my baldness didn't seem to distract my uncle. He was actually looking me in the eyes. Most people couldn't stop their focus from wandering up to my head.

'Yeah, I try to get there whenever I feel well enough.'

'Where's Brett?'

'Brett!' Mum hollered.

Brett strode from his room to where we were gathered in the dining room talking about anything but the real reason for this visit. He was wearing a Metallica t-shirt and was uncharacteristically charming as he shook Uncle Les's hand and then grabbed about four Iced Vovos and stuffed them into his mouth all at once.

'How're the guitar lessons going?' Uncle Les asked Brett.

'Good,' Brett answered, sending flecks of coconut everywhere.

'Go grab your guitar and play something that Kirsty can sing along to.'

Brett stopped chomping.

There's no way he's going to sit down and do a song with me. We aren't the Brady Bunch.

Brett walked off. I waited to hear his bedroom door slam shut. Mum and Dad sipped their tea.

'I can't believe how much you look like your mum,' said Uncle Les.

Really? No one ever says that. They just look at the surface. Mum's colouring is dark, mine has always been light, but maybe we do look alike ...

Then Brett returned with his guitar and a pick. He sat right in front of me and fiddled with the knobs, tuning the strings and strumming a few chords.

I gaped.

'"Save Tonight"?' he asked me, as he swallowed the last of the biscuits. 'Save Tonight' was a single by a singer called Eagle-Eye Cherry, whom Brett had recently introduced me to. My taste in music was moulded by Mum, Dad, Danielle and Brett, who gave me plenty of aural candy to consume. I never felt the urge to go and buy my own music because there were so many different kinds being played at home already. Mum and Dad gifted me The Beatles, Abba, The

Carpenters, Phil Collins and Midnight Oil; Danielle kept me up to date with the latest and greatest of dance and pop; and Brett … he gave me anything with a guitar part that he could teach himself to play.

Stunned, all I could do was nod at Brett.

He began to strum his guitar and, as he did, the screaming of my bones grew quiet. Knowing I needed a cue as to when to start singing the first verse, Brett gave me a very deliberate nod and smiled warmly at me. We sang the whole song and, despite having never performed the song together, we didn't make any mistakes. Uncle Les sat back in his chair, as if our singing had nudged him into relaxation. Dad's lips trembled and red streaks on the whites of his eyes heralded tears. He looked down and fiddled with his empty tea cup. Mum got up and started jostling things about in the kitchen.

Even though I've never felt close to Brett, I saved our song, 'Save Tonight', inside my heart, and I will hold it there forever.

too.' It was my turn to be speechless. 'Your mum's never liked talking about it.'

'And do you talk about it?'

'Yeah ...'

'That's why we don't see you, isn't it?' He didn't answer, but he didn't have to. 'I'd really like it if you could visit.'

'I'd like that too.'

'Can you try?' I asked.

'Sure, darlin'. You promise me you're all right? I know you're very sick.'

'I promise. I was even at school today.'

'Good on you.'

'I better go. Mum will be home soon.'

'Okay. I'm glad you called and hopefully I'll see you soon.'

'Bye, Uncle Les.'

'See you later, sweetheart.'

I hung up.

Oh my goodness! I'm Aboriginal.

* * *

'Mum.' I cornered her as soon as she got home. 'Where are our relatives from?'

'What do you mean? Dad's side of the family is from Scotland and my mum, your grandmother, is Italian.' There was a slight snappiness to Mum's tone.

CHAPTER 35

A Visitor

My Place by Sally Morgan was one of the books I was studying for English for my final exams. As it turned out, Sally Morgan's mum was Aboriginal, but had claimed to be Italian, so it seemed that what my mum had told me about her ancestry was an unoriginal tale. Inside the core of my soul I craved some sort of proof that I was Aboriginal. I wanted something solid. I wanted more than the Kirinari girls calling me 'sister' whenever they kept me company in the school toilets. I wanted more than a conversation on the phone with Uncle Les and his proud wearing of the Aboriginal flag on his t-shirt. I didn't know exactly what I wanted or even how to find it. But until I figured out the answers, I had cancer and end-of-school exams to keep me busy.

Chemo was still hard at work killing my blood, but at least this time I had the assistance of GCSF (granulocyte colony-stimulating factor). GCSF was an injection that wasn't around the first time I had had leukaemia. It was a clever comrade that I developed great affection for. This crafty drug helped your blood cells to grow, and god knows my poor poisoned blood could do with a helping hand. The terrific small syringes of GCSF meant that, during my second dance with cancer, I had to have fewer red blood cell and platelet transfusions. I was also allowed to give these injections to myself. I just had to jab my thigh at home after chemo at hospital. These injections were also the least painful I'd ever had.

We kept the syringes inside the lettuce crisper, because that was the warmest part of the fridge. I wasn't so smart to begin with. When I first got the GCSF injections, I put them on the top shelf of the fridge next to the milk, and minuscule ice cubes formed in the liquid. The colder the contents of an injection, the more it stung — so you can imagine how much this first injection hurt. Dad, being a practical and intelligent man, suggested I pop them inside the lettuce crisper, because the whole point of the crisper was that it was designed to never get icy. I'd then take the syringe out of its home with the lettuce about twenty minutes before I jabbed myself with it.

The exams grew closer. I was doing my best to study and have chemo and not die and give myself GCSF. As marvellous as GCSF was, it didn't always work, so about three weeks out from the exams, Dr Sue did a blood test to make sure I was well enough to sit them. She said she'd call if anything was wrong.

The day of my first exam, English Paper 1, came, and Dr Sue hadn't called. My blood and brain collaborated, and I completed the exam.

Then it was the day of English Paper 2. I woke with a throbbing headache, which squeezed my eyeballs and made them water and ache, but I'd had a headache pretty much every day since my relapse, so I knew I could still sit the exam.

I took some Panadeine Forte a few minutes before the start, but my headache didn't abate. My hand unravelled roads of words onto the exam paper. My heart galloped, but these were my final exams and I was nervous.

Perhaps my headache isn't even a chemo headache. Maybe I have a stress headache like 'normal' teenagers get.

My handwriting became larger and less legible as the two-hour exam unfolded. A sensation of dreaminess overcame me. It felt like the time I was on morphine and a fairy had materialised in the bathtub.

It must be the Panadeine Forte making me feel fuzzy.

'Pens down.'

The exam was over and I'd finished every section. As if on a cloud, I hovered beside my friends as we went to our hang-out spot near the basketball courts to have something to eat. I rummaged in my backpack for my water bottle and my painkillers. The headache was now holding each of my eyeballs inside clenched fists. I swallowed two more pills. Their rancid, metallic taste soiled my tongue and throat.

I pulled out an apple and held it up so one of my friends could take the first bite for me. They were used to this. Chemo gave me agonising jaw pain, which meant even taking the first chomp from an apple was excruciating. Once they had taken a bite for me, I could then nibble my way through the rest of the apple. Jake rolled his eyes as I held out the fruit. Something about this request for assistance always irritated him. Ben took an enormous bite out of my apple while I was still holding it.

'Hey! You ate half of it!'

Ben shrugged and grinned at me with his eyes.

Carefully, I began to take bird-like pecks out of the apple. As I chewed, jarring bolts of pain shot through my jaw. Mother Nature's sugar scalded the inside of my cheeks and the roof of my mouth, and stung my ulcers and bleeding gums (yet more gifts from chemo).

'Here,' I said, handing the apple to Ben, 'I can't eat it.'

'You sure?' he asked.

'Yep, I'm sure.'

He took the apple and finished it in four bites. I was jealous as I watched him devour it, core and all.

'Kirsty!' a voice shrieked from several metres away. It was Mum.

No way. This is so embarrassing.

'Kirsty! Get your bag. We have to go to the hospital right now.' She grabbed my arm and pulled me to my feet.

'Why? What's wrong?'

My friends looked as stunned as I felt.

'You've got no platelets! Dr Sue rang. You have absolutely *no* platelets!'

What does she mean, 'no platelets'?

My platelets often get low — very, very low — but there was never none left at all.

'Okay, okay,' I said casually. I picked up my bag and Mum snatched it from me. She marched off and I followed her, waving goodbye to my friends as I went.

'Did you feel sick before your exam this morning?' snapped Mum. 'Didn't you feel run down or weak or something?!'

Geez, Mum's furious.

'Sort of,' I said.

'This is serious, Kirsty. You've got to stop pushing yourself. I know you want to do everything your friends are doing, but you're not like your friends.'

Wait … she's not angry. She's scared.

'I'm sorry, Mum. I didn't mean to worry you. I swear that all I noticed this morning was that I had a headache, but I've got headaches most of the time, so I didn't think it was anything to worry about.'

She didn't say a word to me the whole way to Randwick. She didn't even listen to Cher.

How could I not know my blood had run out of platelets? How on earth did I do my English exams while running on empty? If Death comes, how will I know it has arrived?

* * *

'How long has she been shaking like this?'

'Since last night.'

'And when did her speech become affected?'

'She seemed to be stuttering and slurring her words a few hours ago, but now ... now she can barely seem to get a word out.'

Dr Sue and Mum looked the most concerned that I'd ever seen either of them.

My hands, arms and legs trembled and shook uncontrollably. Silently, I had tried willing my limbs to be still for several hours, but my body wasn't listening to me — it was demanding we all listen to it. It was trying to tell us something. I'd been topped up to the brim with platelets and thought I'd be going home today, but my body and brain often disagreed with one another.

'My best guess would be that it's some kind of neurological reaction to one of the drugs,' said Dr Sue.

'Neurological?!' Mum's eyes widened. 'You mean the chemo's done something to her brain?'

'That's what it looks like,' said Dr Sue. 'It's probably the Ara-C.'

Ara-C was just one of the many drugs being used in the chemo stew that was meant to help me survive. Ara-C forces cancer cells to take their own lives, but of course, like all chemo drugs, it also caused healthy cells to commit cell suicide. Ara-C was delivered into my body via thigh injections that had the pain-power of a thousand wasp stings.

With a shaky hand, I reached out towards Mum. She knew what I wanted to say and spoke for me.

'She's got some exams left.'

'Kirsty, I can't let you go anywhere,' said Dr Sue. 'We'll have to stop the Ara-C, but I'll need to figure out what to replace it with. I'm not sure what to do about this.'

Dr Sue doesn't know what to do. Shit.

'We'll give you some Valium and hopefully that will stop, or at least help with the shaking.' Valium was a muscle relaxant that was sometimes accompanied by a surge of euphoria. 'The effect on your speech is a real worry. I'm going to have to sleep on this Ara-C …'

'Don't …' I managed to blurt out.

'Don't try to talk, love,' said Mum. 'Just try to relax.'

I dug deep inside myself. There's always more strength to be found as long as you're prepared to get filthy digging for it. I slammed out my words. 'Don't sleep on Ara-C. It'll hurt.' My joke wiped the fear from Mum's and Dr Sue's faces. Dr Sue even laughed. I'd never heard her laugh before. It was a fluttery, fear-filled exhalation, but it was still a laugh all the same.

* * *

For a few days, I was in trembling limbo — literally and metaphorically. As the Ara-C faded from my body, I continued to shake uncontrollably and could barely formulate a word at a time. Dr Sue was still figuring out what on earth she was going to do with me. How would she continue to treat me if we removed Ara-C from my treatment protocol? Scott, the nurse with the piercings who had built Matthew's space station, came in to give me some Valium to relax my muscles and give me a slight reprieve from my shocking shakes.

'Did you hear?' he said. 'Olivia Newton-John is visiting the ward tomorrow.'

'Oh my gosh!' gushed Mum. 'That's incredible. Kirsty and I love her! Isn't that exciting, love?'

Meet someone I idolise with a face cursed with steroid-induced red pustules? Meet one of the most talented women I'd ever seen perform with my freakish bald head? Meet Sandy Olsson, while my life perched and wobbled on a tightrope?

'No,' I blurted out. I put my convulsing hands over my face. 'Look bad,' I stammered.

'She's had cancer herself,' Mum reminded me. 'I don't think she'll even bat an eyelid about how you look. You're sick and that's why she's coming to visit the ward.'

I curled up into a ball, keeping my hands over my face. 'No,' I said again.

The Valium soon settled the tremors, so I actually got some sleep that night.

* * *

Whenever famous people came to the ward — actors, musicians, athletes — the parents often seemed more excited than us kids. Mums and dads would line up for their turn in the parent bathroom so they could shower and change out of their comfy trackpants, t-shirts and thongs into jeans and button-up blouses or shirts. Dads would slather on too much cologne and mums would share what little make-up they had brought among themselves. They often all ended up wearing the same lipstick.

I never knew who arranged for these famous people to walk into our world of illness and death, but any distraction from reality was welcomed by all of us.

When Olivia Newton-John arrived at the hospital, I knew at once, because all the nursing staff had suddenly vanished.

'Curtain,' I barked at Mum, meaning I wanted her to pull the curtain around my bed. There's no way I was going to let the star of my favourite movie, *Grease*, see me like this.

Olivia came into the room. I could hear parents talking to her from behind my safe cocoon.

'Can we get an autograph?'

'Is it okay if we take a picture?'

I could hear her angelic voice, but she spoke in hushed tones so her replies were inaudible.

She spent time with every single patient in the room and spoke to all the parents, listening intently to each unique cancer story as it unravelled. I even heard her play a game of Jenga with a patient who was in a bed near the window. No famous person had ever spent this much time in cancer-country before. They usually sped in with their entourage, took an obligatory photograph with any one of us who was bald, and then left as swiftly as they'd arrived. The photo would then appear in a newspaper or a magazine a few days later. Olivia, however, seemed to be hanging around like she had all the time in the world.

Then, just outside the curtain, I heard the delicate voice of Sandy: 'Is there a patient in there?'

Mum went out and closed the curtain behind her, concealing me from this beautiful woman. 'Hi, my name's Jill,' she said.

'Hi Jill, it's lovely to meet you,' said Olivia. 'How are things going today?'

'Well ... things aren't so great. My daughter Kirsty relapsed, so this is her second time with cancer. She needed a transplant, but there wasn't a match, so we've been hitting her with chemo, but she's had a bad neurological reaction to one of her drugs ... Now we don't know what's going to happen. We're waiting for her oncologist to figure out a new plan.'

'I'm so sorry to hear that.' It sounded like Olivia genuinely cared about me and Mum. 'May I speak to Kirsty?'

'Please don't be offended,' explained Mum, 'if she wasn't so sick, she'd be ecstatic to meet you, but the steroids have ruined her face and she's embarrassed for you to see her. Perhaps you could just sign my hospital diary?'

Mum's hospital diary was where she kept a record of every single day I had cancer: every tablet I swallowed, what I ate, when I ate, when my friends called … everything.

Silence. Olivia must have been signing Mum's diary.

I heard the curtain push open a small way and then close. I pulled my hands off my face and opened my eyes.

Olivia Newtown-John was about twenty centimetres away from my ugliness.

I quickly put my hands back over my cheeks.

'Kirsty,' said Olivia.

From the other side of the curtain, Mum called out, 'She's having trouble speaking at the moment because of the neuro damage, but she can hear you.'

'Kirsty,' Olivia said again. 'Do you think you could open your eyes just for a few moments?'

Of course I couldn't possibly say 'no' to her, so I opened my eyes and pulled my hands down, but only slightly. A tear fell from each of my eyes. The salt made my flesh burn. A few more tears fell and made a tiny puddle on my pillow under my right eye.

With smooth, delicate, coconut-scented hands, she gently pulled my hands away from my face. She looked like she hadn't aged a day since *Grease*. Her hair was cut into a sleek blonde bob, her fringe was perfectly straight and there wasn't a single hair out of place. Her eyes shone with empathy. No one had ever looked at me the way she was looking at me right now. More tears descended. I couldn't help it. I tried to stop crying, but I couldn't. She sat with me for several minutes and gently dabbed at my tears with a tissue.

I couldn't believe I was meeting Olivia Newton-John and crying in front of her. She didn't say anything the whole time, and thankfully Mum was on the other side of the curtain or she would've reminded me of her 'no crying' rule. After some time, I seemed to run out of tears.

Thank goodness!

I went to put my hands back over my face, but she clasped my wrists determinedly and stopped me. Then she spoke: 'You're going to get through this.' Her words, like her hands, were delicate and determined. She said it again: 'Kirsty, you're going to get through this.'

She was the beauty, but she had no qualms about being right up close to the face of the beast. Jake liked to keep a two-metre distance between us because of how disgusting he thought my appearance was, but here was the most stunning woman I'd ever met and she was so close to me I could smell the spearmint freshness of her breath. She had even touched my hands without hesitation. 'You're going to get through this,' she said a third and final time. She stood up, kissed my forehead and left.

Perhaps she was right. Perhaps I could get through this and perhaps I needed to stop worrying so much about what I looked like.

And there was no 'perhaps' about something else — Olivia Newton-John was the kindest and most empathetic visitor to ever walk among the ward. If only all our celebrity guests could have been more like her.

* * *

It took days for the tremors to stop, and my words came back into my mouth, but they got twisted and tangled if I didn't speak slowly and carefully pronounce each syllable.

Dr Sue replaced Ara-C with lots of extra methotrexate, which meant more lumbar punctures, more tablets and more intravenous treatment.

I missed two of my final exams. That meant I wouldn't graduate with my friends and I wouldn't get my marks the same day they did. I'd have to do the exams I missed next year through TAFE or distance education.

I still attended graduation day. I came first in Drama, English and Ancient History.

Will I survive next year — the third year of chemotherapy? Will the chemo even work? If I live long enough to get into university, I want to go to the University of Sydney. I liked how it felt there when I was going to Patti's writing classes. It's also one of the hardest universities to get into and if I'm going to go to university, I may as well aim for the best.

* * *

My body endured my third and final year of chemo. A year after graduation, arrangements were made for me to sit my exams at home under the supervision of a little old lady sent by the Department of Education. For three years my body had been infiltrated with drugs, violated with countless injections, witnessed death after death of children and even had Death breathe its foul-smelling breath too close to my face. But somehow, I persevered.

I survived.

I survived.

I was 19 years old and I had survived cancer twice.

CHAPTER 36

Anything Is Possible

My exam results had arrived in the mail. I held the envelope in my hands and turned it over again and again.

'What are you waiting for?' said Mum. 'Open it, love.'

I slowly slid my finger through the paper of the envelope and pulled out an A4-sized document. My name and address were clearly printed with my student number at the top of the page, and right underneath was my UAI — my total score for all my subjects, out of one hundred.

Oh my gosh … 98.88.

'What did you get?' asked Mum.

I couldn't speak, so I shoved the piece of paper at her.

She looked at it. 'Oh my god! Call your father!'

I called Dad and told him.

'Congratulations. I'm so proud of you,' he said. 'A mark like that is an amazing achievement for any student, but to get it and to have gone through what you've gone through at the same time … it's remarkable. What do you think you want to do?'

'I don't know, Dad,' I said, and I really didn't. I had absolutely no idea. I'd never thought about what kind of job or career I'd like to have when I was a grown-up because I think part of me was afraid I would not make it into the world of adulthood. 'I know I want to go to the University of Sydney. I applied for a few things there. Maybe I'll do a Bachelor of Arts degree, because then I can study all kinds of subjects and it might help me figure out the kind of job I want.' I didn't mention to him, nor to anyone else, that I wasn't confident my body would stay in remission, so I didn't feel any pressure to pick a career path.

'That sounds like a smart idea to me,' said Dad. 'I would've loved to have done an arts degree. I'll see you tonight and you'd better have a hug waiting for me, all right?'

'Yes, Dad.'

When it came time to select my subjects, I decided to study anything that sounded interesting to me: Philosophy, Sociology, Psychology, Anthropology, English (of course), as well as Performance Studies and Aboriginal Studies. Mum might not be offering up any knowledge about our family's Aboriginal ancestry, but surely one of the best universities in Australia would have the information I required.

* * *

Before I started my degree, there was one more fundraising event that I needed to attend. But this one was a little different to all the others. I arranged this one.

The 'Kirsty's Finished Chemo Party' was the name my family and I gave to the event. It was a gathering with a small cover charge, the proceeds of which would go to the Children's Cancer Institute of Australia. We booked out a function space with a bar, and we hired a DJ. We invited pretty much everyone we knew to come and eat, drink and remember that even though I was the embodiment of some people's worst nightmares, I was also someone who proved that the impossible was within reach. Surely being a miracle personified was reason to celebrate.

A few hundred people came. Danielle wrote me a poem especially for the occasion and read it out loud for everybody to hear:

Three years has passed since that bastard 'cancer',
Decided to come back for more.
We thought it had left us years ago;
What was it looking for?

Whatever it wanted, it didn't get
Because it came to the wrong place.
Kirsty kicked your arse, cancer,
So stick that in your face.

From the very start of her relapse,
Kirsty put everyone first.
She worried about friends and family,
When she was feeling her absolute worst.

There is no one I know with her strength
To survive what she's been through.
If it had happened to any of us,
We wouldn't have known what to do.

But Kirst fought on and she always will;
Nothing can get in her way.
She's our inspirational fairy,
And we'd die if she wasn't here today.

* * *

I walked along my very own 'yellow-brick road' (though the tiles on the ground were actually a rusty red) to the Koori Centre Library in the Old Teachers' College at the University of Sydney. Magpies cried out to me from outside the arch-shaped windows. My thongs flapped on my feet, and I nervously reached up to fondle a piece of my shoulder-length blonde hair. Sometimes I needed to remind myself I wasn't a bald freak any more. I chewed anxiously on a piece of spearmint-flavoured chewing gum. Sometimes

I could still taste the chemo tablets or the acetone flavour of vincristine.

I felt like all I'd been through had heightened my senses — or was it my appreciation of existence that had been heightened? Did the green tops of trees against the clear blue sky look as vivid to everyone else as they did to me? Did anyone notice the perfume left behind after someone had mown the grass as much as I did? Did the waxiness of a Pink Lady apple feel as good against anyone's skin as it did to me?

Crickets frolicked in my tummy as I wandered around the Old Teachers' College, looking for the library. I decided to go to the bathroom first, and then renew my search.

As I washed my hands, a young woman came out of one of the cubicles and began washing her hands next to me. I smiled at her in the mirror and she smiled back like she knew an embarrassing secret about me. Mischief shone out of her brown eyes. I looked down at my hideously white arms. Mine were the arms of a girl who had sat intimately alongside Death. Her healthy arms were the same Milo colour as Matt's and Mum's arms.

She continued beaming at me, so I said, 'Hey.'

'Hey, sister. Now, you look *a lot* better than the last time I saw you in the dunnies.'

I *knew* this young woman. 'Oh my gosh! You went to my high school! Your name's Daisy.'

'Yep.'

'You had a huge crush on Tyson!'

She laughed from deep inside at the mention of Tyson. 'Yeah, well, he was the hottest blackfella at Kirinari. All of us girls had crushes on him. What are you doing here?'

'I'm headed to the Koori Centre Library. I'm doing a Bachelor of Arts and one of the subjects I chose is Aboriginal Studies.'

'Cool! I'm doing an Arts degree too. Want me to show you where the library is, sister?'

'Yeah, that would be great.'

It was the smallest library I'd ever been to in my entire life. It was packed with books from the floor to the ceiling. The tables and chairs had stacks of books piled on them.

How will I find anything in here — especially when I don't know what I'm looking for?

Then a bright-yellow book on the top of a stack caught my eye. There were old black-and-white photos on the front cover. I recognised one of them. I'd seen it before, when rummaging through Mum's secret stash of photos. It was a photo of my Mum's grandmother. She looked just like *my* grandmother, Mum's mum, who'd died long before I was born. I picked up the book. It was called *The Darug and their Neighbours* by James Kohen.

'What is it?' asked Daisy.

'That's my great-grandmother.'

I began frantically flicking through the pages. The book contained the names of all my ancestors, listed one after the other. My insides sprang joyfully to life as I stopped on page 156. At the top of the page, there it was: 'Kirsty Everett'.

'Oh my gosh! My name's in here.'

'Why do you look so surprised, sister?'

'I don't know.'

'Surely you knew you were Koori. We told you! I guess your Mum can't deny it now.'

'Well … she can and probably will.'

'You don't know that. She might come around one day. Never say never, sister. You never know what might be possible.'

'Yeah … you're right. Maybe anything *is* possible.'

* * *

Mum, Dad and I walked into the red building that housed the Belvoir Street Theatre. I was twenty-one years old, a two-time cancer survivor and a university student. We'd been here before; it was our favourite theatre in Sydney. I'd performed here a couple of times in the downstairs theatre, and we'd come along to all sorts of performances here while I was on chemo the second time. Imagination, art, creativity — whatever label you feel comfortable with — I believe played a part in getting me through my illness — both times. Books I read, artworks I saw, and performances I watched or played a part in, all allowed me to escape from the realm of cancer and death. The brilliance of authors, artists, musicians and actors on a stage or screen were distractions from the pain — sometimes they even allowed me to express and expel the pain. Songs could reduce me to tears — which I always hid from Mum — and songs could also empower me, lift me up, and make me feel like I could be as strong as an ancient Spartan warrior princess.

But today, Dad and I were using the theatre for a different purpose.

'What's this play called again?' asked Mum. Blindly, she'd placed her trust in my selection of the play that the three of us would attend on this Saturday afternoon.

'It's called *Box the Pony*. It's a one-woman show. The actor's name's Leah Purcell and the play is loosely based on her life. She co-wrote the script as well. She's had an interesting life. Her father was a boxer, I think.' My shoulders squeezed up to my ears slightly as I spoke. Nervous adrenaline increased my blood pressure.

'Sounds good,' said Mum.

Dad and I exchanged a quick glance.

We took our seats, which were only two metres away from the small square stage. One of the reasons I liked this theatre was because you were so close to the performers and the tiered seats meant no audience member could obstruct my view of the action onstage (a rarity, considering my small stature). The lights faded to blackout and then came back up to reveal the remarkable Leah Purcell alone onstage.

For the next two hours, Leah told us multiple stories about her life and the lives of her family members as Aboriginals growing up on a mission in Queensland. She had every audience member glued to her the entire time. We hung on every word. We were hypnotised by the fluid movements of her body on stage. We would've all kept watching for an additional two hours.

After the performance, as Leah took a bow, the audience went mental. The applause wouldn't stop. A force beyond my control had me stand up, cup my hands around my mouth and release my appreciation in the form of, 'Woooooooo!' I continued to clap so hard my hands were stinging, but I didn't care. Then Dad stood up. He placed his thumb and index finger in his mouth and did a loud collection of whistles. One by one, other audience members began to stand up as well. Leah's eyes brimmed with tears of joy. Mum remained seated.

Eventually, Leah left the stage while the applause continued and then faded. Then all the lights came up on the stage and in the audience and there was an announcement: 'Ladies and gentlemen, thank you for attending this afternoon's performance of *Box the Pony*. Leah will have a brief amount of time to come out and greet the audience before she needs to get ready for her evening show. She'd like to invite members of the audience to remain behind if they'd like to say "hello" to her.'

'Mum! We've gotta stay,' I urged. 'We might get to meet her!'

'All right,' said Mum.

I was astonished at her lack of resistance.

* * *

'Hey sister, were you the young lady who stood up first in the audience?'

I couldn't believe it. Leah Purcell was standing right in front of me and talking to me. I almost couldn't reply.

'Yeah, that was me,' I replied sheepishly while my insides exploded with ecstasy. 'This is my mum and my dad.'

She shook Dad's hand.

'That was fantastic,' said Dad, who seemed to be blushing.

'Ah, thanks. I'm glad you enjoyed the show. And Mum' — Leah grabbed Mum's hand and shook it — 'what did you think of the show?'

'Oh, you were absolutely marvellous. I don't know how you remember all those lines,' said Mum.

Leah laughed. 'Neither do I sometimes,' she said.

'You know, I'm Aboriginal too,' said Mum. The loud rumblings of the crowded foyer were silenced and my ears began ringing. I felt Dad grab hold of my hand and grip it tightly. My heart thundered inside my ribs.

She's admitted it. I can't believe it. Mum has finally admitted she's Aboriginal.

287

'Yeah, I thought so,' said Leah. 'You and your daughter look similar.'

That's what Uncle Les said!

'Well, I've got to keep moving, but thanks for coming to the show and I'm glad you enjoyed it,' said Leah and off she went. It took a few moments for my sense of hearing to return to normal.

'Should we head home?' asked Dad. All I could do was nod.

I had a thousand questions to ask Mum, but I didn't want to hit her with them today. I felt like a pile of rocks that had been crushing my lungs for years had finally been lifted. I replayed Mum's words in my head over and over again on the car ride home: 'You know, I'm Aboriginal too.'

And so am I. I'm Aboriginal. I'm a blonde-haired, blue-eyed, Aboriginal two-time cancer survivor, and life couldn't be any better.

Life AC (After Cancer)

'When was the last time you had a blood test?' asked Dr John Glenburn.

I shrugged. 'I don't know.'

'When was the last time you went to see Dr Sue Russell?'

'Hmmm … I can't remember. I figure if it was really that important, they'd call me and insist I come in.'

He shook his head, but he wasn't angry with me. Dr John Glenburn, or 'Johnny boy' as I like to call him, is my GP. He's one of the best doctors I've ever known. He plays guitar and wears multi-coloured socks with no shoes in his office, but the best thing about him is that he's incredibly empathetic. He's one of the rare few that have found a way to do his job and maintain a strong, caring sense of humanity — a characteristic so often missing from the registrars that crossed my path as a child.

He's fifty years old but could easily pass for forty. He has photographs in his office of himself surfing on gigantic waves. Whenever I'm in the waiting room, there are always a few senior ladies talking about him. I like to tell him what they say about him: 'Isn't Dr Glenburn's Scottish accent sexy?' He always blushes and grins and says, 'Yes, I'm very popular among the old ladies.'

'All right, how about we do one blood test a year?'

'If you want. That's cool with me.'

'Is there anything that you're worried about? How are the migraines and back pain?'

'I'm not worried I'll get cancer ever again, if that's what you mean. And the migraines and back pain … they're an inconvenience, but I can live with them. I'd rather be alive and occasionally in pain than dead. I figure the pain is a small price to pay and it's no wonder I have it … I mean, they put a lot of drugs in my body to keep me alive. A migraine every now and then, my spine feeling like it has been hit with a sledgehammer — I can handle it.'

'Okay, we'll just take some blood then.' He printed off the blue pathology form and I read the words printed in black:

FBC and LFT
History: Relapsed ALL

FBC stands for Full Blood Count and LFT stands for Liver Function Test. ALL stands for acute lymphoblastic leukaemia.

I couldn't believe my medical history could be summarised in one word and one acronym.

The results came back as normal, as I knew they would. But even though the test results said 'normal', I know blood doesn't always tell the truth.

Sometimes I don't feel like I'm normal, but I've looked into this and most people don't. 'Normal' is probably my least favourite word because I don't think it exists, and trying to be 'normal' seems to cause a lot of trouble for a lot of people. Unless it's in relation to a blood test, then the word 'normal' can go and sit in a distant corner far, far away from me and everybody else it torments.

* * *

'Today we're going to begin to learn about one of the coolest writers and best plays ever written,' I announced to the class. 'We're going to study *Macbeth* by William Shakespeare. Now, a lot of people say they don't like Shakespeare, but it's only because they don't understand it. I promise you, if you understand him, and I'm going to show you how, it's very unlikely that you'll dislike him. We're also going to be learning how to write essays.'

'Ah, Miss ... not essays,' exclaimed one of my Year 9 students.

'Essays are just like Shakespeare. People who don't like them usually don't know how to write them. They're not as bad as everyone thinks. I'm going to show you how I used to write essays when I was at school and university and, as you know, I'm a big English nerd, so if you follow my simple instructions, you'll be able to get really high marks.' I started handing out copies of *Macbeth*. 'The most important thing to keep in mind is that Shakespeare's plays are meant to be performed. You're not supposed to read them alone and you're not supposed to read them sitting down in a chair. You've gotta get up and perform the words.'

'Hey Miss, how come you're really into all this?'

'Words are magic and anyone who doesn't love to read is missing out on something very special. Now, I need three volunteers to get up for the first scene of *Macbeth*. Let's do this!'

ACKNOWLEDGMENTS

I would like to acknowledge my incredible husband, my lover of many lifetimes including this one, Benjamin Malesev. He bought me my first laptop in total faith that I'd be capable of writing this book. There's no way I would've been able to get through this project without him. Thank you so much, my darling.

I'd like to thank his parents, Annette and Steve Malesev, the best in-laws anyone could ask for. They've been supportive throughout this process alongside their remarkable son and I feel privileged and blessed to have married into this family.

Thank you to Patti Miller and the NSW Writers Centre. Patti — you were the first person to tell me I should and could write a book. I'm overjoyed that you were right.

I want to thank Caroline Baum for being the first person to read my work and tell me I'm a writer and for her role as my unofficial guide through the unfamiliar labyrinth of publishing a memoir.

I want to thank my agent, Jeanne Ryckmans, my publisher, Mary Rennie, one of the coolest 'Normies' I've met, and

HarperCollins. Thank you for believing in me and my work and helping me tick off one of the most challenging items on my bucket list.

Thank you to the Children's Cancer Institute of Australia for your ongoing work and to Dr Sue Russell for keeping my body alive when the odds were not in our favour on more than one occasion.

Finally, to cancer, you do far more than just suck and you should never be described as a gift — fuck you and thank you.

ABOUT THE AUTHOR

Kirsty Everett defied the odds and survived two bouts of cancer, aged nine and sixteen. She completed her HSC, as well as a Bachelor of Arts with a double major in English and Aboriginal Studies at the University of Sydney. In addition, she also completed a Bachelor of Teaching so she could teach English and Drama to high-school students.

She has been a motivational and educational speaker since the age of fourteen. Her public speaking for the purpose of helping others with cancer was kickstarted by Professor Darcy O'Gorman-Hughes (who helped establish the Children's Cancer Institute of Australia). In 2006, Kirsty received an award for Outstanding Voluntary Service from NSW Governor Marie Bashir.

Kirsty is now living 'happily ever after' with her husband, and continues to encourage others to support the work of the CCIA.

She always checks the bathroom for fairies.